Table of Contents

Message From the Secretaries vii

Acknowledgments viii

Executive Summary x

Introduction 1

Nutrition & Health Are Closely Related 2

The *Dietary Guidelines for Americans*: What It Is, What It Is Not 5

Developing the *Dietary Guidelines for Americans* 6

    Stage 1: Review of Current Scientific Evidence 7

    Stage 2: Development of the *Dietary Guidelines for Americans* 8

    Stage 3: Implementing the *Dietary Guidelines for Americans* 10

A Roadmap to the 2015-2020 Edition of the *Dietary Guidelines for Americans* 11

Chapter 1. Key Elements of Healthy Eating Patterns 13

Introduction 14

About This Chapter 14

Key Recommendations: Components of Healthy Eating Patterns 15

Healthy Eating Patterns: Dietary Principles 16

The Science Behind Healthy Eating Patterns 17

    Associations Between Eating Patterns & Health 17

    Associations Between Dietary Components & Health 17

A Closer Look Inside Healthy Eating Patterns 18

    Food Groups 21

    Other Dietary Components 28

Examples of Other Healthy Eating Patterns 35

    Healthy Mediterranean-Style Eating Pattern 35

    Healthy Vegetarian Eating Pattern 36

Summary 36

Chapter 2. Shifts Needed To Align With Healthy Eating Patterns 37

Introduction 38

About This Chapter 38

Current Eating Patterns in the United States 38

A Closer Look at Current Intakes & Recommended Shifts 43

    Food Groups 43

    Other Dietary Components 53

    Underconsumed Nutrients & Nutrients of Public Health Concern 60

    Beverages 61

Opportunities for Shifts in Food Choices 61

Summary 62

Chapter 3. Everyone Has a Role in Supporting Healthy Eating Patterns 63

Introduction 64

About This Chapter 64

Creating & Supporting Healthy Choices 64

The Social-Ecological Model 64

    Sectors 65

    Settings 66

    Social & Cultural Norms & Values 66

    Individual Factors 66

Meeting People Where They Are: Contextual Factors & Healthy Eating Patterns 67

    Food Access 67

    Household Food Insecurity 67

    Acculturation 67

Strategies for Action 68

Summary 72

Appendixes

Appendix 1. *Physical Activity Guidelines for Americans* 73

Appendix 2. Estimated Calorie Needs per Day, by Age, Sex, & Physical Activity Level 77

Appendix 3. USDA Food Patterns: Healthy U.S.-Style Eating Pattern 79

Appendix 4. USDA Food Patterns: Healthy Mediterranean-Style Eating Pattern 83

Appendix 5. USDA Food Patterns: Healthy Vegetarian Eating Pattern 86

Appendix 6. Glossary of Terms 89

Appendix 7. Nutritional Goals for Age-Sex Groups Based on Dietary Reference Intakes
& *Dietary Guidelines* Recommendations 97

Appendix 8. Federal Resources for Information on Nutrition & Physical Activity 99

Appendix 9. Alcohol 101

Appendix 10. Food Sources of Potassium 104

Appendix 11. Food Sources of Calcium 108

Appendix 12. Food Sources of Vitamin D 111

Appendix 13. Food Sources of Dietary Fiber 114

Appendix 14. Food Safety Principles & Guidance 119

List of Tables

Table I-1. Facts About Nutrition- & Physical Activity-Related Health Conditions in the United States 2

Table 1-1. Healthy U.S.-Style Eating Pattern at the 2,000-Calorie Level, With Daily or
Weekly Amounts From Food Groups, Subgroups, & Components 18

Table 1-2. Composition of the Healthy Mediterranean-Style & Healthy Vegetarian Eating Patterns
at the 2,000-Calorie Level, With Daily or Weekly Amounts From Food Groups, Subgroups, & Components 35

Table 2-1. Examples of Vegetables in Each Vegetable Subgroup 47

Table A1-1. *Physical Activity Guidelines for Americans* Recommendations 73

Table A1-2. Federal Physical Activity Resources 75

Table A2-1. Estimated Calorie Needs per Day, by Age, Sex, & Physical Activity Level 77

Table A3-1. Healthy U.S.-Style Eating Pattern: Recommended Amounts of Food
From Each Food Group at 12 Calorie Levels 80

Table A4-1. Healthy Mediterranean-Style Eating Pattern: Recommended Amounts of Food
From Each Food Group at 12 Calorie Levels 84

Table A5-1. Healthy Vegetarian Eating Pattern: Recommended Amounts of Food
From Each Food Group at 12 Calorie Levels 87

Table A6-1. Body Mass Index & Corresponding Body Weight Categories for Children & Adults 89

Table A7-1. Daily Nutritional Goals for Age-Sex Groups Based on Dietary Reference Intakes
& *Dietary Guidelines* Recommendations 97

Table A8-1. Federal Nutrition & Physical Activity Resources 99

Table A9-1. Alcoholic Drink-Equivalents of Select Beverages 102

Table A10-1. Potassium: Food Sources Ranked by Amounts of Potassium & Energy
per Standard Food Portions & per 100 Grams of Foods 104

Table A11-1. Calcium: Food Sources Ranked by Amounts of Calcium & Energy
per Standard Food Portions & per 100 Grams of Foods 108

Table A12-1. Vitamin D: Food Sources Ranked by Amounts of Vitamin D & Energy
per Standard Food Portions & per 100 Grams of Foods 111

Table A13-1. Dietary Fiber: Food Sources Ranked by Amounts of Dietary Fiber
and Energy per Standard Food Portions & per 100 Grams of Foods 114

Table A14-1. Recommended Safe Minimum Internal Temperatures 121

List of Figures

Figure ES-1. *2015-2020 Dietary Guidelines for Americans* at a Glance xv

Figure I-1. Adherence of the U.S. Population Ages 2 Years & Older to the *2010 Dietary Guidelines*,
as Measured by Average Total Healthy Eating Index-2010 (HEI-2010) Scores 4

Figure I-2. Percentage of Adults Meeting the *Physical Activity Guidelines*
(Aerobic & Muscle-Strengthening Recommendations) 5

Figure I-3. Science, Policy, Implementation: Developing the *2015-2020 Dietary Guidelines for Americans* 6

Figure 1-1. Cup- & Ounce-Equivalents 19

Figure 1-2. Fatty Acid Profiles of Common Fats & Oils 26

Figure 1-3. Hidden Components in Eating Patterns 29

Figure 2-1. Dietary Intakes Compared to Recommendations. Percent of the
U.S. Population Ages 1 Year & Older Who Are Below, At, or Above Each Dietary Goal or Limit................... 39

Figure 2-2. Empower People To Make Healthy Shifts 40

Figure 2-3. Average Daily Food Group Intakes by Age-Sex Groups, Compared to Ranges of Recommended Intake 41

Figure 2-4. Average Vegetable Subgroup Intakes in Cup-Equivalents per Week by Age-Sex Groups,
Compared to Ranges of Recommended Intakes per Week 44

Figure 2-5. Average Whole & Refined Grain Intakes in Ounce-Equivalents per Day by Age-Sex Groups,
Compared to Ranges of Recommended Daily Intake for Whole Grains & Limits for Refined Grains 48

Figure 2-6. Average Protein Foods Subgroup Intakes in Ounce-Equivalents
per Week by Age-Sex Groups, Compared to Ranges of Recommended Intake 50

Figure 2-7. Average Intakes of Oils & Solid Fats in Grams per Day by Age-Sex
Group, in Comparison to Ranges of Recommended Intake for Oils 52

Figure 2-8. Typical Versus Nutrient-Dense Foods & Beverages 53

Figure 2-9. Average Intakes of Added Sugars as a Percent of Calories per Day by Age-Sex Group,
in Comparison to the *Dietary Guidelines* Maximum Limit of Less Than 10 Percent of Calories 54

Figure 2-10. Food Category Sources of Added Sugars in the U.S. Population Ages 2 Years & Older 55

Figure 2-11. Average Intakes of Saturated Fats as a Percent of Calories per Day by Age-Sex Group,
in Comparison to the *Dietary Guidelines* Maximum Limit of Less Than 10 Percent of Calories 56

Figure 2-12. Food Category Sources of Saturated Fats in the U.S. Population Ages 2 Years & Older 57

Figure 2-13. Average Intakes of Sodium in Milligrams per Day by Age-Sex Groups,
Compared to Tolerable Upper Intake Levels (UL) 58

Figure 2-14. Food Category Sources of Sodium in the U.S. Population Ages 2 Years & Older 59

Figure 3-1. A Social-Ecological Model for Food & Physical Activity Decisions 65

Figure 3-2. Implementation of the *Dietary Guidelines* Through MyPlate 69

Figure 3-3. Strategies To Align Settings With the *2015-2020 Dietary Guidelines for Americans* 70

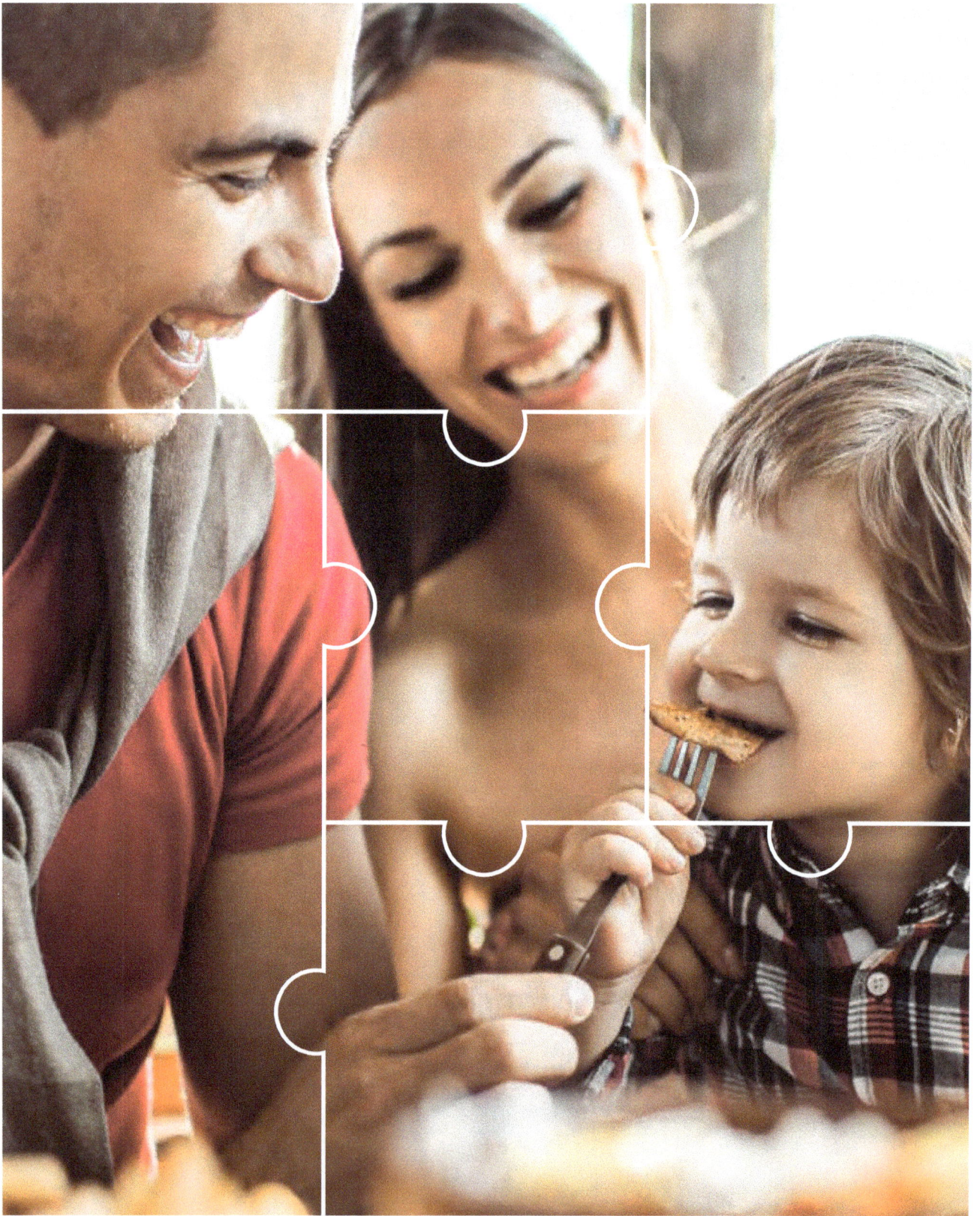

Message From the Secretaries

One of our Government's most important responsibilities is to protect the health of the American public. Today, about half of all American adults—117 million people—have one or more preventable, chronic diseases, many of which are related to poor quality eating patterns and physical inactivity. Rates of these chronic, diet-related diseases continue to rise, and they come not only with increased health risks, but also at high cost. In 2008, the medical costs linked to obesity were estimated to be $147 billion. In 2012, the total estimated cost of diagnosed diabetes was $245 billion, including $176 billion in direct medical costs and $69 billion in decreased productivity.

The *Dietary Guidelines for Americans* is an essential resource for health professionals and policymakers as they design and implement food and nutrition programs that feed the American people, such as USDA's National School Lunch Program and School Breakfast Program, which feed more than 30 million children each school day. The *Dietary Guidelines* also provides information that helps Americans make healthy choices for themselves and their families.

This new edition of the *Dietary Guidelines*, the *2015-2020 Dietary Guidelines for Americans*, is grounded in the most current scientific evidence and is informed by the recommendations of the 2015 Dietary Guidelines Advisory Committee. This Federal advisory committee, which was composed of prestigious researchers in the fields of nutrition, health, and medicine, conducted a multifaceted, robust process to analyze the available body of scientific evidence. Their work culminated in a scientific report which provided advice and recommendations to the Federal Government on the current state of scientific evidence on nutrition and health. Informed by this report and by consideration of public and Federal agency comments, HHS and USDA nutrition and health experts then developed the *Dietary Guidelines*.

The *2015-2020 Dietary Guidelines* provides guidance for choosing a healthy diet and focuses on preventing the diet-related chronic diseases that continue to affect our population. Its recommendations are ultimately intended to help individuals improve and maintain overall health and reduce the risk of chronic disease. Its focus is disease prevention, not treatment. This edition also includes data describing the significant differences between Americans' current consumption and the *Dietary Guidelines* recommendations. It also recommends where shifts are encouraged to help people achieve healthy eating patterns. These analyses will assist professionals and policymakers as they use the *Dietary Guidelines* to help Americans adopt healthier eating patterns and make healthy choices in their daily lives, while enjoying food and celebrating cultural and personal traditions through food. Now more than ever, we recognize the importance of focusing not on individual nutrients or foods in isolation, but on everything we eat and drink—healthy eating patterns as a whole—to bring about lasting improvements in individual and population health.

The body of scientific literature looking at healthy eating patterns and their impact on disease prevention is far more robust now than ever before. Chronic diet-related diseases continue to rise and levels of physical activity remain low. Progress in reversing these trends will require comprehensive and coordinated strategies, and the *Dietary Guidelines* is an important part of a complex and multifaceted solution to promote health and help to reduce the risk of chronic disease. The *Dietary Guidelines* translates science into succinct, food-based guidance that can be relied upon to help Americans choose a healthy eating pattern and enjoyable diet. We believe that aligning with the recommendations in the *Dietary Guidelines* will help many Americans lead healthier and more active lives.

/Sylvia M. Burwell/

Sylvia M. Burwell
Secretary, U.S. Department of
Health and Human Services

/Thomas J. Vilsack/

Thomas J. Vilsack
Secretary, U.S. Department
of Agriculture

USDA

Acknowledgments

The U.S. Department of Health and Human Services and the U.S. Department of Agriculture acknowledge the work of the 2015 Dietary Guidelines Advisory Committee whose recommendations informed revisions for this edition of the *Dietary Guidelines for Americans*.

Dietary Guidelines Advisory Committee Members

Barbara Millen, DrPH, RD; Alice H. Lichtenstein, DSc; Steven Abrams, MD; Lucile Adams-Campbell, PhD; Cheryl Anderson, PhD, MPH; J. Thomas Brenna, PhD; Wayne Campbell, PhD; Steven Clinton, MD, PhD; Gary Foster, PhD (May–August 2013); Frank Hu, MD, PhD, MPH; Miriam Nelson, PhD; Marian Neuhouser, PhD, RD; Rafael Pérez-Escamilla, PhD; Anna Maria Siega-Riz, PhD; Mary Story, PhD, RD. Consultants: Timothy S. Griffin, PhD; Michael W. Hamm, PhD; Michael G. Perri, PhD, ABPP.

The Departments also acknowledge the work of the departmental scientists, staff, and policy officials responsible for the production of this document.

Policy Officials

HHS: Karen B. DeSalvo, MD, MPH, MSc; Howard K. Koh, MD, MPH; Don Wright, MD, MPH.

USDA: Kevin W. Concannon, MSW; Angela Tagtow, MS, RD, LD; Jackie Haven, MS, RD.

Policy Document Writing Staff

Richard Olson, MD, MPH; Kellie Casavale, PhD, RD; Colette Rihane, MS, RD; Eve Essery Stoody, PhD; Patricia Britten, PhD; Jill Reedy, PhD, MPH, RD; Elizabeth Rahavi, RD; Janet de Jesus, MS, RD; Katrina Piercy, PhD, RD; Amber Mosher, MPH, RD; Stephenie Fu; Jessica Larson, MS, RD; Anne Brown Rodgers (Editor).

Policy Document Reviewers/Technical Assistance

The Departments acknowledge the contributions of numerous other internal departmental scientists who provided consultation and extensive review throughout the production of this document. Additionally, the Departments acknowledge the external, independent peer reviewers for their work to ensure technical accuracy in the translation of the science into policy.

Finally, the Departments would like to acknowledge the important role of those who provided public comments throughout this process.

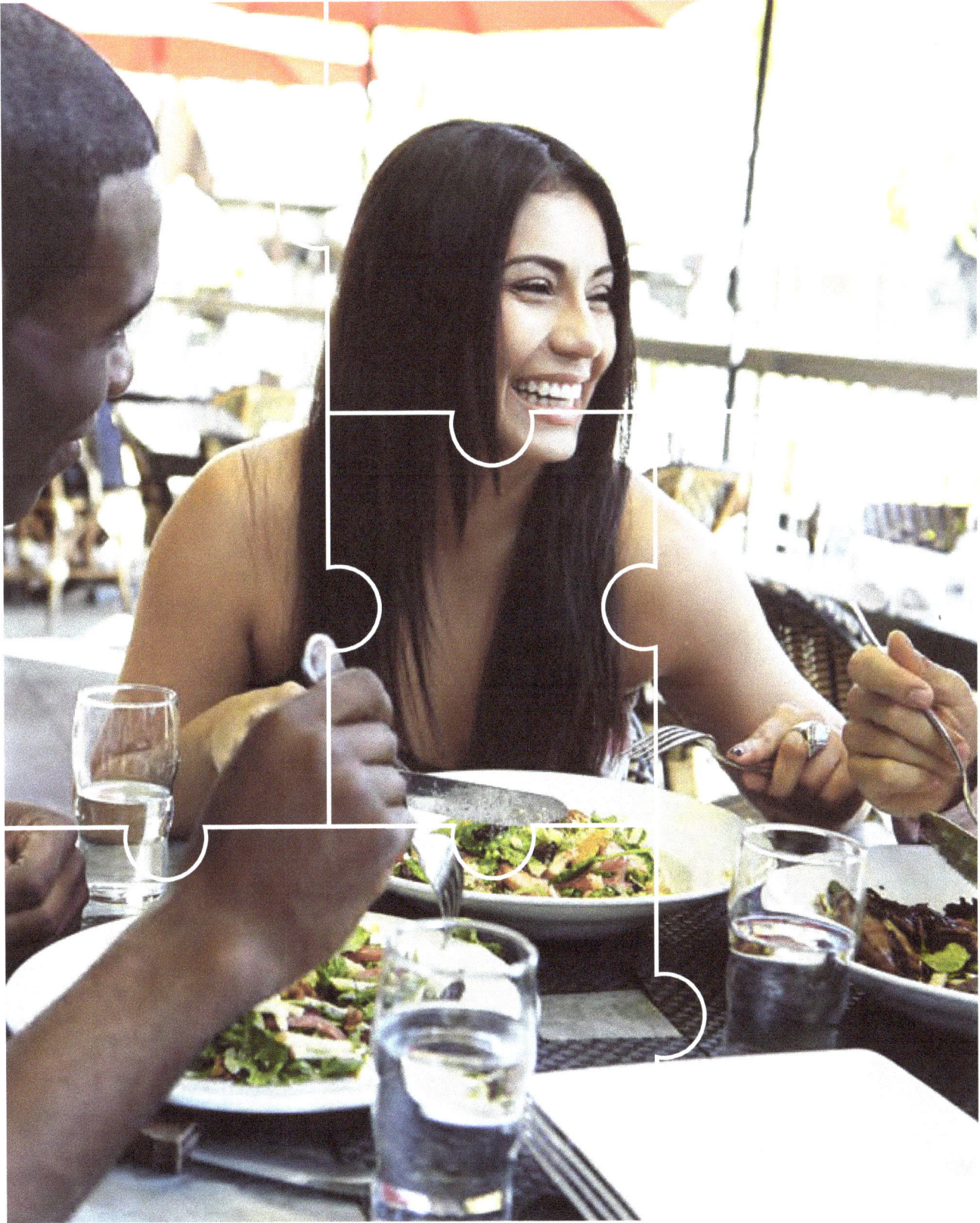

Executive Summary

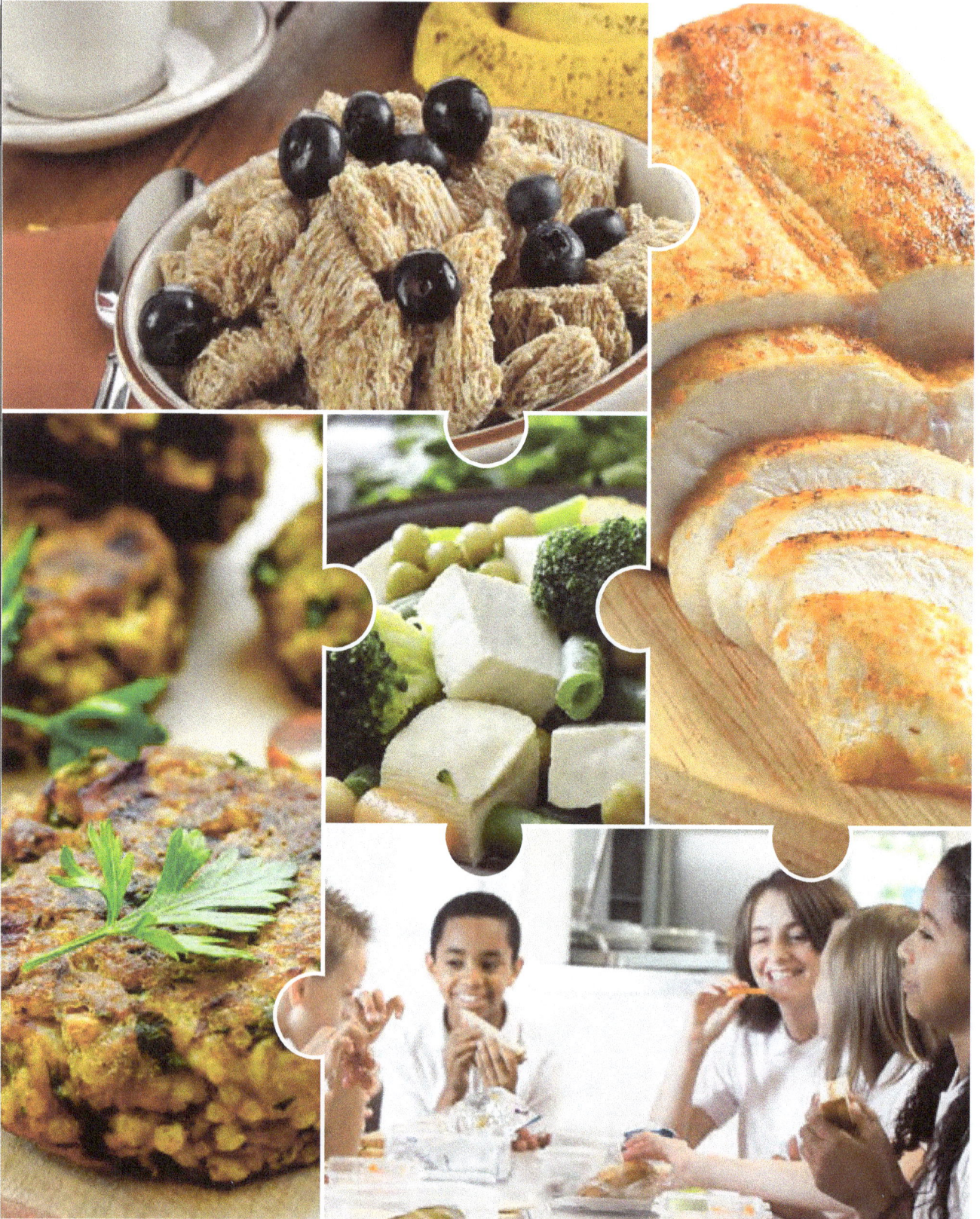

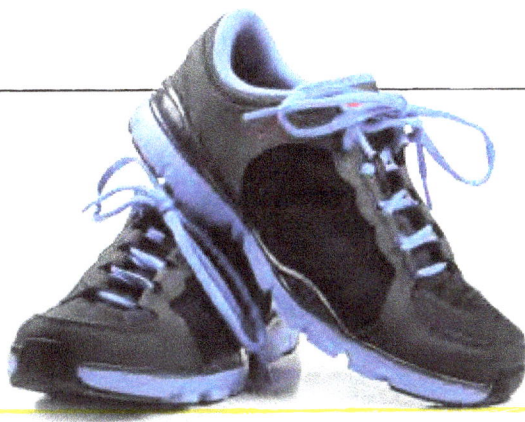

Over the past century, deficiencies of essential nutrients have dramatically decreased, many infectious diseases have been conquered, and the majority of the U.S. population can now anticipate a long and productive life. At the same time, rates of chronic diseases—many of which are related to poor quality diet and physical inactivity—have increased. About half of all American adults have one or more preventable, diet-related chronic diseases, including cardiovascular disease, type 2 diabetes, and overweight and obesity.

However, a large body of evidence now shows that healthy eating patterns and regular physical activity can help people achieve and maintain good health and reduce the risk of chronic disease throughout all stages of the lifespan. The *2015-2020 Dietary Guidelines for Americans* reflects this evidence through its recommendations.

The *Dietary Guidelines* is required under the 1990 National Nutrition Monitoring and Related Research Act, which states that every 5 years, the U.S. Departments of Health and Human Services (HHS) and of Agriculture (USDA) must jointly publish a report containing nutritional and dietary information and guidelines for the general public. The statute (Public Law 101-445, 7 U.S.C. 5341 et seq.) requires that the *Dietary Guidelines* be based on the preponderance of current scientific and medical knowledge. The 2015-2020 edition of the *Dietary Guidelines* builds from the 2010 edition with revisions based on the *Scientific Report of the 2015 Dietary Guidelines Advisory Committee* and consideration of Federal agency and public comments.

The *Dietary Guidelines* is designed for professionals to help all individuals ages 2 years and older and their families consume a healthy, nutritionally adequate diet. The information in the *Dietary Guidelines* is used in developing Federal food, nutrition, and health policies and programs. It also is the basis for Federal nutrition education materials designed for the public and for the nutrition education components of HHS and USDA food programs. It is developed for use by policymakers and nutrition and health professionals. Additional audiences who may use *Dietary Guidelines* information to develop programs, policies, and communication for the general public include businesses, schools, community groups, media, the food industry, and State and local governments.

Previous editions of the *Dietary Guidelines* focused primarily on individual dietary components such as food groups and nutrients. However, people do not eat food groups and nutrients in isolation but rather in combination, and the totality of the diet forms an overall eating pattern. The components of the eating pattern can have interactive and potentially cumulative effects on health. These patterns can be tailored to an individual's personal preferences, enabling Americans to choose the diet that is right for them. A growing body of research has examined the relationship between overall eating patterns, health, and risk of chronic disease, and findings on these relationships are sufficiently well established to support dietary guidance. As a result, eating patterns and their food and nutrient characteristics are a focus of the recommendations in the *2015-2020 Dietary Guidelines*.

The *2015-2020 Dietary Guidelines* provides five overarching Guidelines that encourage healthy eating patterns, recognize that individuals will need to make shifts in their food and beverage choices to achieve a healthy pattern, and acknowledge that all segments of our society have a role to play in supporting healthy choices. These Guidelines also embody the idea that a healthy eating pattern is not a rigid prescription, but rather, an adaptable framework in which individuals can enjoy foods that meet their personal, cultural, and traditional preferences and fit within their budget. Several examples of healthy eating patterns that translate and integrate the recommendations in overall healthy ways to eat are provided.

The Guidelines

1 **Follow a healthy eating pattern across the lifespan.** All food and beverage choices matter. Choose a healthy eating pattern at an appropriate calorie level to help achieve and maintain a healthy body weight, support nutrient adequacy, and reduce the risk of chronic disease.

2 **Focus on variety, nutrient density, and amount.** To meet nutrient needs within calorie limits, choose a variety of nutrient-dense foods across and within all food groups in recommended amounts.

3 **Limit calories from added sugars and saturated fats and reduce sodium intake.** Consume an eating pattern low in added sugars, saturated fats, and sodium. Cut back on foods and beverages higher in these components to amounts that fit within healthy eating patterns.

4 **Shift to healthier food and beverage choices.** Choose nutrient-dense foods and beverages across and within all food groups in place of less healthy choices. Consider cultural and personal preferences to make these shifts easier to accomplish and maintain.

5 **Support healthy eating patterns for all.** Everyone has a role in helping to create and support healthy eating patterns in multiple settings nationwide, from home to school to work to communities.

Key Recommendations provide further guidance on how individuals can follow the five Guidelines. The *Dietary Guidelines'* Key Recommendations for healthy eating patterns should be applied in their entirety, given the interconnected relationship that each dietary component can have with others.

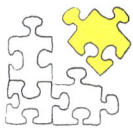

Key Recommendations:

Consume a healthy eating pattern that accounts for all foods and beverages within an appropriate calorie level.

A healthy eating pattern includes:[1]

- A variety of vegetables from all of the subgroups—dark green, red and orange, legumes (beans and peas), starchy, and other
- Fruits, especially whole fruits
- Grains, at least half of which are whole grains
- Fat-free or low-fat dairy, including milk, yogurt, cheese, and/or fortified soy beverages
- A variety of protein foods, including seafood, lean meats and poultry, eggs, legumes (beans and peas), and nuts, seeds, and soy products
- Oils

A healthy eating pattern limits:

- Saturated fats and *trans* fats, added sugars, and sodium

Key Recommendations that are quantitative are provided for several components of the diet that should be limited. These components are of particular public health concern in the United States, and the specified limits can help individuals achieve healthy eating patterns within calorie limits:

- Consume less than 10 percent of calories per day from added sugars[2]
- Consume less than 10 percent of calories per day from saturated fats[3]
- Consume less than 2,300 milligrams (mg) per day of sodium[4]
- If alcohol is consumed, it should be consumed in moderation—up to one drink per day for women and up to two drinks per day for men—and only by adults of legal drinking age.[5]

In tandem with the recommendations above, Americans of all ages—children, adolescents, adults, and older adults—should meet the *Physical Activity Guidelines for Americans* to help promote health and reduce the risk of chronic disease. Americans should aim to achieve and maintain a healthy body weight. The relationship between diet and physical activity contributes to calorie balance and managing body weight. As such, the *Dietary Guidelines* includes a Key Recommendation to:

- Meet the *Physical Activity Guidelines for Americans.*[6]

[1] Definitions for each food group and subgroup are provided throughout Chapter 1: Key Elements of Healthy Eating Patterns and are compiled in Appendix 3. USDA Food Patterns: Healthy U.S.-Style Eating Pattern.

[2] The recommendation to limit intake of calories from added sugars to less than 10 percent per day is a target based on food pattern modeling and national data on intakes of calories from added sugars that demonstrate the public health need to limit calories from added sugars to meet food group and nutrient needs within calorie limits. The limit on calories from added sugars is not a Tolerable Upper Intake Level (UL) set by the Institute of Medicine (IOM). For most calorie levels, there are not enough calories available after meeting food group needs to consume 10 percent of calories from added sugars and 10 percent of calories from saturated fats and still stay within calorie limits.

[3] The recommendation to limit intake of calories from saturated fats to less than 10 percent per day is a target based on evidence that replacing saturated fats with unsaturated fats is associated with reduced risk of cardiovascular disease. The limit on calories from saturated fats is not a UL set by the IOM. For most calorie levels, there are not enough calories available after meeting food group needs to consume 10 percent of calories from added sugars and 10 percent of calories from saturated fats and still stay within calorie limits.

[4] The recommendation to limit intake of sodium to less than 2,300 mg per day is the UL for individuals ages 14 years and older set by the IOM. The recommendations for children younger than 14 years of age are the IOM age- and sex-appropriate ULs (see Appendix 7. Nutritional Goals for Age-Sex Groups Based on Dietary Reference Intakes and Dietary Guidelines Recommendations).

[5] It is not recommended that individuals begin drinking or drink more for any reason. The amount of alcohol and calories in beverages varies and should be accounted for within the limits of healthy eating patterns. Alcohol should be consumed only by adults of legal drinking age. There are many circumstances in which individuals should not drink, such as during pregnancy. See Appendix 9. Alcohol for additional information.

[6] U.S. Department of Health and Human Services. *2008 Physical Activity Guidelines for Americans.* Washington (DC): U.S. Department of Health and Human Services; 2008. ODPHP Publication No. U0036. Available at: http://www.health.gov/paguidelines. Accessed August 6, 2015.

Terms To Know

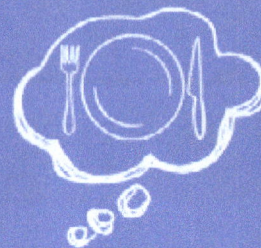

Several terms are used to operationalize the principles and recommendations of the *2015-2020 Dietary Guidelines*. These terms are essential to understanding the concepts discussed herein:

Eating Pattern—The combination of foods and beverages that constitute an individual's complete dietary intake over time. Often referred to as a "dietary pattern," an eating pattern may describe a customary way of eating or a combination of foods recommended for consumption. Specific examples include USDA Food Patterns and the Dietary Approaches to Stop Hypertension (DASH) Eating Plan.

Nutrient Dense—A characteristic of foods and beverages that provide vitamins, minerals, and other substances that contribute to adequate nutrient intakes or may have positive health effects, with little or no solid fats and added sugars, refined starches, and sodium. Ideally, these foods and beverages also are in forms that retain naturally occurring components, such as dietary fiber. All vegetables, fruits, whole grains, seafood, eggs, beans and peas, unsalted nuts and seeds, fat-free and low-fat dairy products, and lean meats and poultry—when prepared with little or no added solid fats, sugars, refined starches, and sodium—are nutrient-dense foods. These foods contribute to meeting food group recommendations within calorie and sodium limits. The term "nutrient dense" indicates the nutrients and other beneficial substances in a food have not been "diluted" by the addition of calories from added solid fats, sugars, or refined starches, or by the solid fats naturally present in the food.

Variety—A diverse assortment of foods and beverages across and within all food groups and subgroups selected to fulfill the recommended amounts without exceeding the limits for calories and other dietary components. For example, in the vegetables food group, selecting a variety of foods could be accomplished over the course of a week by choosing from all subgroups, including dark green, red and orange, legumes (beans and peas), starchy, and other vegetables.

An underlying premise of the *Dietary Guidelines* is that nutritional needs should be met primarily from foods. All forms of foods, including fresh, canned, dried, and frozen, can be included in healthy eating patterns. Foods in nutrient-dense forms contain essential vitamins and minerals and also dietary fiber and other naturally occurring substances that may have positive health effects. In some cases, fortified foods and dietary supplements may be useful in providing one or more nutrients that otherwise may be consumed in less-than-recommended amounts.

For most individuals, achieving a healthy eating pattern will require changes in food and beverage choices. This edition of the *Dietary Guidelines* focuses on shifts to emphasize the need to make substitutions—that is, choosing nutrient-dense foods and beverages in place of less healthy choices—rather than increasing intake overall. Most individuals would benefit from shifting food choices both within and across food groups. Some needed shifts are minor and can be accomplished by making simple substitutions, while others will require greater effort to accomplish.

Although individuals ultimately decide what and how much to consume, their personal relationships; the settings in which they live, work, and shop; and other contextual factors strongly influence their choices. Concerted efforts among health professionals, communities, businesses and industries, organizations, governments, and other segments of society are needed to support individuals and families in making dietary and physical activity choices that align with the *Dietary Guidelines*. Everyone has a role, and these efforts, in combination and over time, have the potential to meaningfully improve the health of current and future generations.

Figure ES-1.
2015-2020 Dietary Guidelines for Americans at a Glance

The *2015-2020 Dietary Guidelines* focuses on the big picture with recommendations to help Americans make choices that add up to an overall healthy eating pattern. To build a healthy eating pattern, combine healthy choices from across all food groups—while paying attention to calorie limits, too. Check out the 5 Guidelines that encourage healthy eating patterns:

1

Follow a healthy eating pattern across the lifespan. All food and beverage choices matter. Choose a healthy eating pattern at an appropriate calorie level to help achieve and maintain a healthy body weight, support nutrient adequacy, and reduce the risk of chronic disease.

Follow a healthy eating pattern over time to help support a healthy body weight and reduce the risk of chronic disease.

A Healthy Eating Pattern Includes:

Fruits Vegetables Protein

Dairy Grains Oils

A Healthy Eating Pattern Limits:

Saturated Fats & *Trans* Fats Added Sugars Sodium

2

Focus on variety, nutrient density, and amount. To meet nutrient needs within calorie limits, choose a variety of nutrient-dense foods across and within all food groups in recommended amounts.

Choose a variety of nutrient-dense foods from each food group in recommended amounts.

Example Meal:

Lettuce & Celery — Vegetables Grains — Whole-Grain Bread

Apples & Grapes — Fruits Dairy — Fat-Free Milk

Chicken Breast & Unsalted Walnuts — Protein Oils — Mayonnaise

2015-2020 Dietary Guidelines for Americans at a Glance

The *2015-2020 Dietary Guidelines* focuses on the big picture with recommendations to help Americans make choices that add up to an overall healthy eating pattern. To build a healthy eating pattern, combine healthy choices from across all food groups—while paying attention to calorie limits, too. Check out the 5 Guidelines that encourage healthy eating patterns:

3

Limit calories from added sugars and saturated fats and reduce sodium intake. Consume an eating pattern low in added sugars, saturated fats, and sodium. Cut back on foods and beverages higher in these components to amounts that fit within healthy eating patterns.

Consume an eating pattern low in added sugars, saturated fats, and sodium.

Example Sources of:

Added Sugars

Saturated Fats

Sodium

4

Shift to healthier food and beverage choices. Choose nutrient-dense foods and beverages across and within all food groups in place of less healthy choices. Consider cultural and personal preferences to make these shifts easier to accomplish and maintain.

Replace typical food and beverages choices with more nutrient-dense options. Be sure to consider personal preferences to maintain shifts over time.

Example:

Shift

Meal A

Meal B

Everyone has a role in helping to create and support healthy eating patterns in places where we learn, work, live, and play.

5

Support healthy eating patterns for all. Everyone has a role in helping to create and support healthy eating patterns in multiple settings nationwide, from home to school to work to communities.

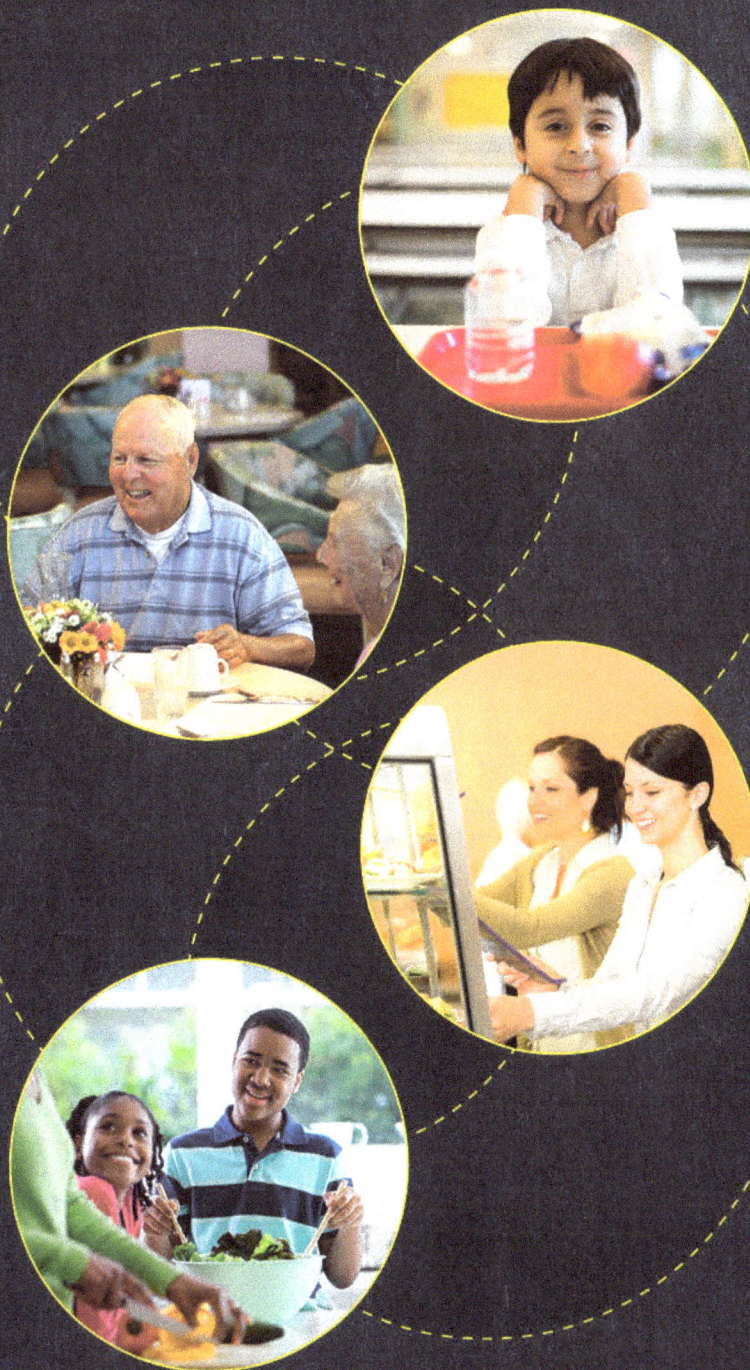

Introduction

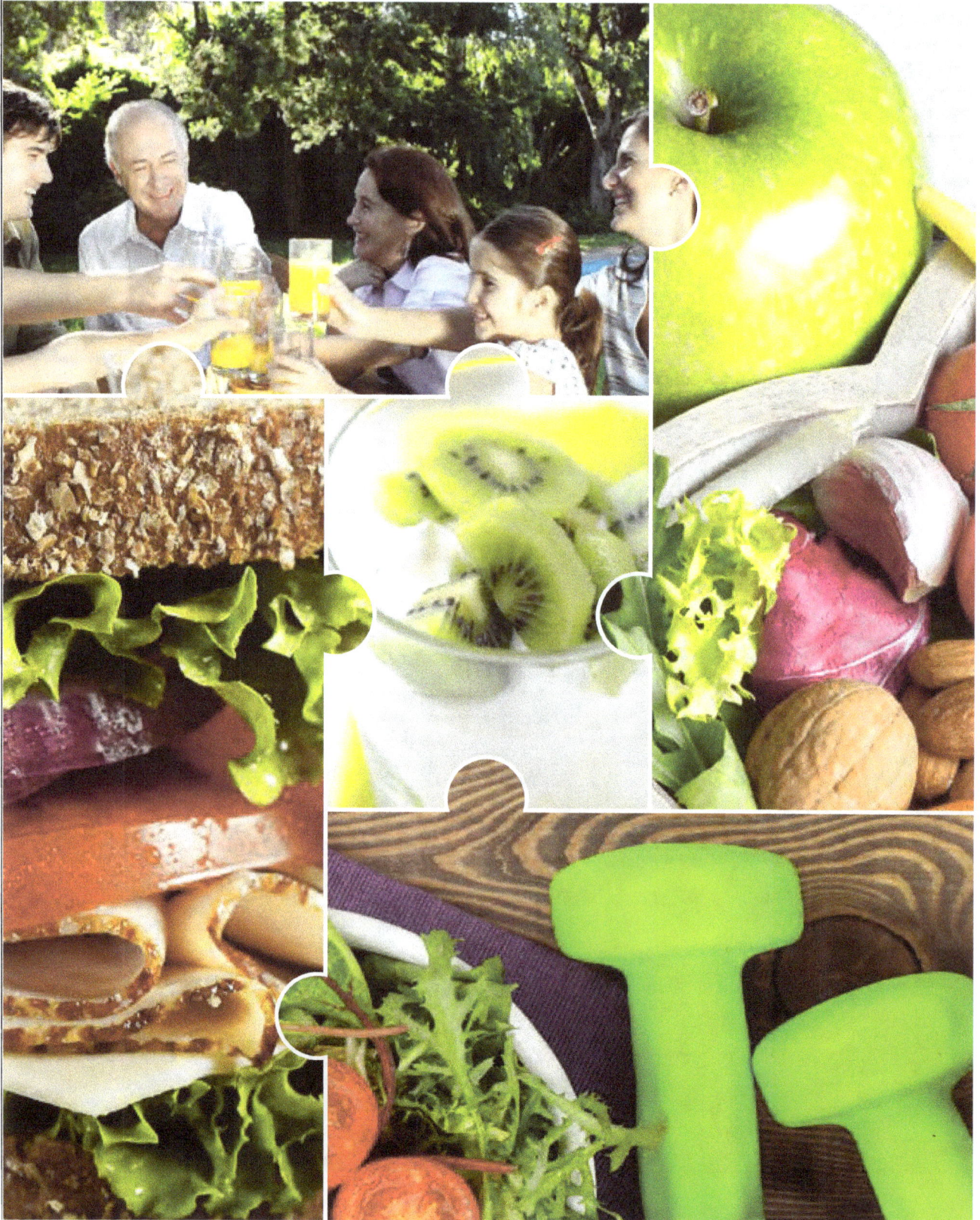

Every 5 years since 1980, a new edition of the *Dietary Guidelines for Americans* has been published. Its goal is to make recommendations about the components of a healthy and nutritionally adequate diet to help promote health and prevent chronic disease for current and future generations. Although many of its recommendations have remained relatively consistent over time, the *Dietary Guidelines* has evolved as scientific knowledge has grown. These advancements have provided a greater understanding of, and focus on, the importance of healthy eating patterns as a whole, and how foods and beverages act synergistically to affect health. Therefore, healthy eating patterns is a focus of the *2015-2020 Dietary Guidelines*.

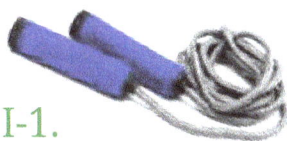

Nutrition & Health Are Closely Related

Over the past century, essential nutrient deficiencies have dramatically decreased, many infectious diseases have been conquered, and the majority of the U.S. population can now anticipate a long and productive life. However, as infectious disease rates have dropped, the rates of noncommunicable diseases—specifically, chronic diet-related diseases—have risen, due in part to changes in lifestyle behaviors. A history of poor eating and physical activity patterns have a cumulative effect and have contributed to significant nutrition- and physical activity-related health challenges that now face the U.S. population. About half of all American adults—117 million individuals—have one or more preventable chronic diseases, many of which are related to poor quality eating patterns and physical inactivity. These include cardiovascular disease, high blood pressure, type 2 diabetes, some cancers, and poor bone health. More than two-thirds of adults and nearly one-third of children and youth are overweight or obese. These high rates of overweight and obesity and chronic disease have persisted for more than two decades and come not only with increased health risks, but also at high cost. In 2008, the medical costs associated with obesity were estimated to be $147 billion. In 2012, the total estimated cost of diagnosed diabetes was $245 billion, including $176 billion in direct medical costs and $69 billion in decreased productivity.[1]

Table I-1 describes the high rates of nutrition- and physical activity-related chronic diseases and their related risk factors. These diseases affect all ages—children, adolescents, adults, and older adults—though rates vary by several factors, including race/ethnicity, income status, and body weight status.

Table I-1.

Facts About Nutrition & Physical Activity-Related Health Conditions in the United States

Health Condition	Facts
Overweight & Obesity	<ul><li>For more than 25 years, more than half of the adult population has been overweight or obese.</li><li>Obesity is most prevalent in those ages 40 years and older and in African American adults, and is least prevalent in adults with highest incomes.</li><li>Since the early 2000s, abdominal obesity[a] has been present in about half of U.S. adults of all ages. Prevalence is higher with increasing age and varies by sex and race/ethnicity.</li><li>In 2009-2012, 65% of adult females and 73% of adult males were overweight or obese.</li><li>In 2009-2012, nearly one in three youth ages 2 to 19 years were overweight or obese.</li></ul>

[1] For more information, see: Centers for Disease Control and Prevention (CDC). Chronic Disease Overview. August 26, 2015. Available at http://www.cdc.gov/chronicdisease/overview/. Accessed November 3, 2015.

Table I-1. *(continued...)*

Facts About Nutrition & Physical Activity-Related Health Conditions in the United States

Health Condition	Facts
Cardiovascular Disease (CVD) & Risk Factors: Coronary Heart Disease Stroke Hypertension High Total Blood Cholesterol	• In 2010, CVD affected about 84 million men and women ages 20 years and older (35% of the population). • In 2007-2010, about 50% of adults who were normal weight, and nearly three-fourths of those who were overweight or obese, had at least one cardiometabolic risk factor (i.e., high blood pressure, abnormal blood lipids, smoking, or diabetes). • Rates of hypertension, abnormal blood lipid profiles, and diabetes are higher in adults with abdominal obesity. • In 2009-2012, almost 56% of adults ages 18 years and older had either prehypertension (27%) or hypertension (29%).[b] • In 2009-2012, rates of hypertension among adults were highest in African Americans (41%) and in adults ages 65 years and older (69%). • In 2009-2012, 10% of children ages 8 to 17 years had either borderline hypertension (8%) or hypertension (2%).[c] • In 2009-2012, 100 million adults ages 20 years or older (53%) had total cholesterol levels ≥200 mg/dL; almost 31 million had levels ≥240 mg/dL. • In 2011-2012, 8% of children ages 8 to 17 years had total cholesterol levels ≥200 mg/dL.
Diabetes	• In 2012, the prevalence of diabetes (type 1 plus type 2) was 14% for men and 11% for women ages 20 years and older (more than 90% of total diabetes in adults is type 2). • Among children with type 2 diabetes, about 80% were obese.
Cancer[d]: Breast Cancer Colorectal Cancer	• Breast cancer is the third leading cause of cancer death in the United States. • In 2012, an estimated 3 million women had a history of breast cancer. • Colorectal cancer is the second leading cause of cancer death in the United States. • In 2012, an estimated 1.2 million adult men and women had a history of colorectal cancer.
Bone Health	• A higher percent of women are affected by osteoporosis (15%) and low bone mass (51%) than men (about 4% and 35%, respectively). • In 2005-2010, approximately 10 million (10%) adults ages 50 years and older had osteoporosis and 43 million (44%) had low bone mass.

[a] Abdominal obesity, as measured by waist circumference, is defined as a waist circumference of >102 centimeters in men and >88 centimeters in women.

[b] For adults, prehypertension was defined as a systolic blood pressure of 120-139 mm mercury (Hg) or diastolic blood pressure of 80-89 mm Hg among those who were not currently being treated for hypertension. Hypertension was defined as systolic blood pressure (SBP) >140 mm Hg, diastolic blood pressure (DBP) >90 mm Hg, or taking antihypertensive medication.

[c] For children, borderline hypertension was defined as systolic or diastolic blood pressure at the 90th percentile or higher but lower than the 95th percentile or as blood pressure levels of 120/80 mm Hg or higher (but less than the 95th percentile). Hypertension was defined as a systolic or diastolic blood pressure at the 95th percentile or higher.

[d] The types of cancer included here are not a complete list of all diet- and physical activity-related cancers.

Concurrent with these diet-related health problems persisting at high levels, trends in food intake over time show that, at the population level, Americans are not consuming healthy eating patterns. For example, the prevalence of overweight and obesity has risen and remained high for the past 25 years, while Healthy Eating Index (HEI) scores, a measure of how food choices align with the *Dietary Guidelines*, have remained low (**Figure I-1**). Similarly, physical activity levels have remained low over time (**Figure I-2**). The continued high rates of overweight and obesity and low levels of progress toward meeting *Dietary Guidelines* recommendations highlight the need to improve dietary and physical activity education and behaviors across the U.S. population. Progress in reversing these trends will require comprehensive and coordinated strategies, built on the *Dietary Guidelines* as the scientific foundation, that can be maintained over time. The *Dietary Guidelines* is an important part of a complex and multifaceted solution to promoting health and helping to reduce the risk of chronic disease.

Figure I-1.

Adherence of the U.S. Population Ages 2 Years and Older to the *2010 Dietary Guidelines*, as Measured by Average Total Healthy Eating Index-2010 (HEI-2010) Scores

■ Maximum Total Score

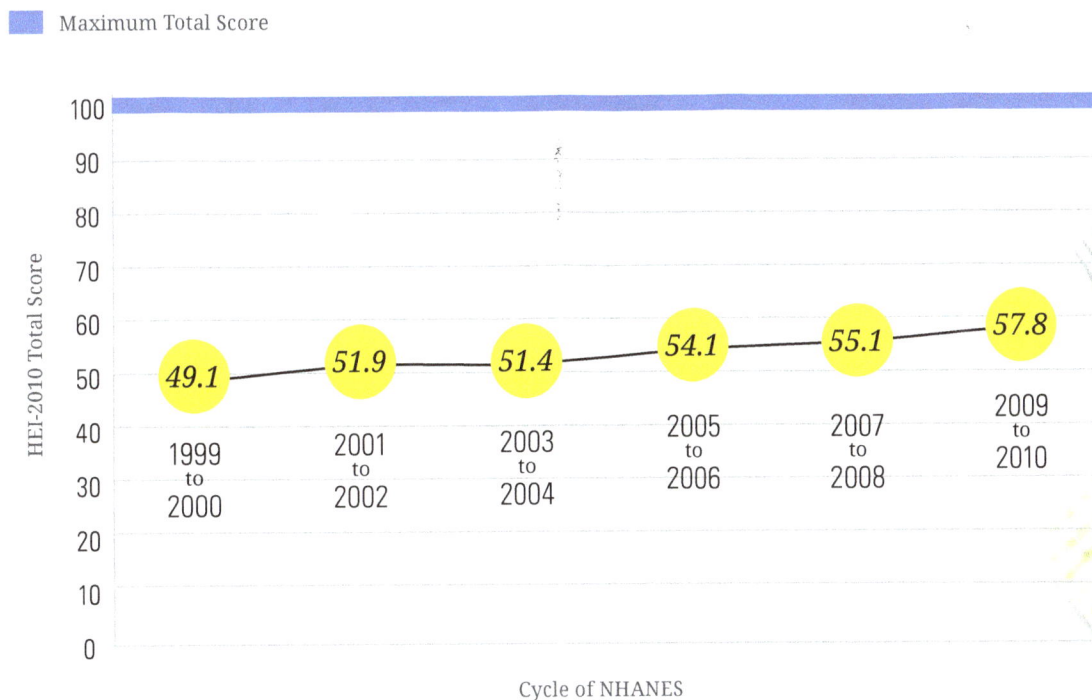

DATA SOURCES: Analyses of What We Eat in America, National Health and Nutrition Examination Survey (NHANES) data from 1999-2000 through 2009-2010.

NOTE: HEI-2010 total scores are out of 100 possible points. A score of 100 indicates that recommendations on average were met or exceeded. A higher total score indicates a higher quality diet.

Figure I-2.
Percentage of Adults Meeting the *Physical Activity Guidelines* (Aerobic & Muscle-Strengthening Recommendations)

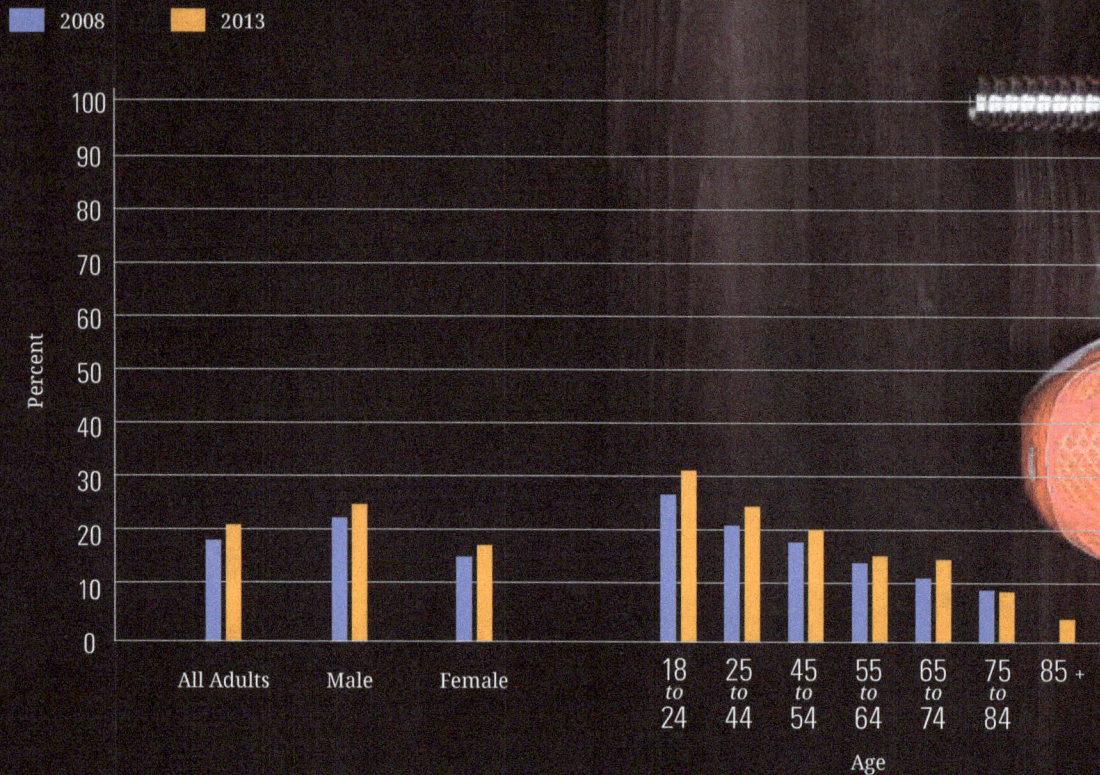

Legend: ■ 2008 ■ 2013

Y-axis: Percent (0, 10, 20, 30, 40, 50, 60, 70, 80, 90, 100)

X-axis categories: All Adults, Male, Female, 18 to 24, 25 to 44, 45 to 54, 55 to 64, 65 to 74, 75 to 84, 85 +

Age

DATA SOURCES: Analyses of the National Health Interview Survey, 2008 and 2013.
Healthy People 2020 PA-2.4. Increase the proportion of adults who meet the objectives for aerobic physical activity and for muscle strengthening activity. Washington, DC: U.S. Department of Health and Human Services, Office of Disease Prevention and Health Promotion, June 3, 2015. Available at: http://www.healthypeople.gov/2020/data-search/Search-the-Data?nid=5072.

The *Dietary Guidelines for Americans*: What It Is, What It Is Not

The main purpose of the *Dietary Guidelines* is to inform the development of Federal food, nutrition, and health policies and programs. The primary audiences are policymakers, as well as nutrition and health professionals, not the general public. The *Dietary Guidelines* is a critical tool for professionals to help Americans make healthy choices in their daily lives to help prevent chronic disease and enjoy a healthy diet. It serves as the evidence-based foundation for nutrition education materials that are developed by the Federal Government for the public. For example, Federal dietary guidance publications are required by law to be consistent with the *Dietary Guidelines*. It also is used to inform USDA and HHS food programs, such as USDA's National School Lunch Program and School Breakfast Program, which feed more than 30 million children each school day, and the Special Supplemental Nutrition Program for Women, Infants and Children, which uses the *Dietary Guidelines* as the scientific underpinning for its food packages and nutrition education program with about 8 million beneficiaries. In HHS, the Administration on Aging implements the *Dietary Guidelines* through the Older Americans Act Nutrition Services programs (i.e., nutrition programs for older adults), with about 5,000 community-based nutrition service providers who together serve more

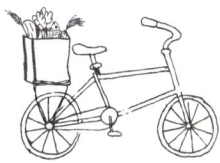

The Importance of Physical Activity in a Healthy Lifestyle

Although the primary focus of the *Dietary Guidelines* is on nutrition recommendations, physical activity is mentioned throughout this edition because of its critical and complementary role in promoting good health and preventing disease, including many diet-related chronic diseases. The following chapters note the role of physical activity in improving health and reducing chronic disease risk; describe the gap between current physical activity recommendations and reported levels of activity; and discuss how the settings in which people live, learn, work, and play can be enhanced to encourage increased physical activity. For more information, see the *Physical Activity Guidelines for Americans* at www.health.gov/paguidelines.

than 900,000 meals a day across the United States. Other Departments, such as the Department of Defense and the Department of Veterans Affairs, also use the *Dietary Guidelines* to inform programs. The *Dietary Guidelines* also may be used to inform the development of programs, policies, and communication by audiences other than the document's principal audiences. These audiences, who share the common goal of serving the general public, include businesses, schools, community groups, media, the food industry, and State and local governments.

The *2015-2020 Dietary Guidelines* translates science into succinct, food-based guidance that can be relied upon to help Americans choose foods that provide a healthy and enjoyable diet. Its recommendations are ultimately intended to help individuals improve and maintain overall health and reduce the risk of chronic disease—its focus is disease prevention. The *Dietary Guidelines* is not intended to be used to treat disease. Regardless of an individual's current health

status, almost all people in the United States could benefit from shifting choices to better support healthy eating patterns. Thus, the *Dietary Guidelines* may be used or adapted by medical and nutrition professionals to encourage healthy eating patterns to patients.

Developing the *Dietary Guidelines for Americans*

A greater understanding of the relationships between nutrition and human health has and will continue to evolve over time. Creating each edition of the *Dietary Guidelines* is a joint effort of HHS and USDA. A new edition is published every 5 years to reflect advancements in scientific knowledge and translate the science current at the time into sound food-based guidance to promote health in the United States.[2] The process to develop the *Dietary Guidelines* has also evolved and includes three stages.

Figure I-3.

Science, Policy, Implementation: Developing the *2015-2020 Dietary Guidelines for Americans*

To develop each edition of the *Dietary Guidelines for Americans*, HHS and USDA collaborate during a 3-stage process.

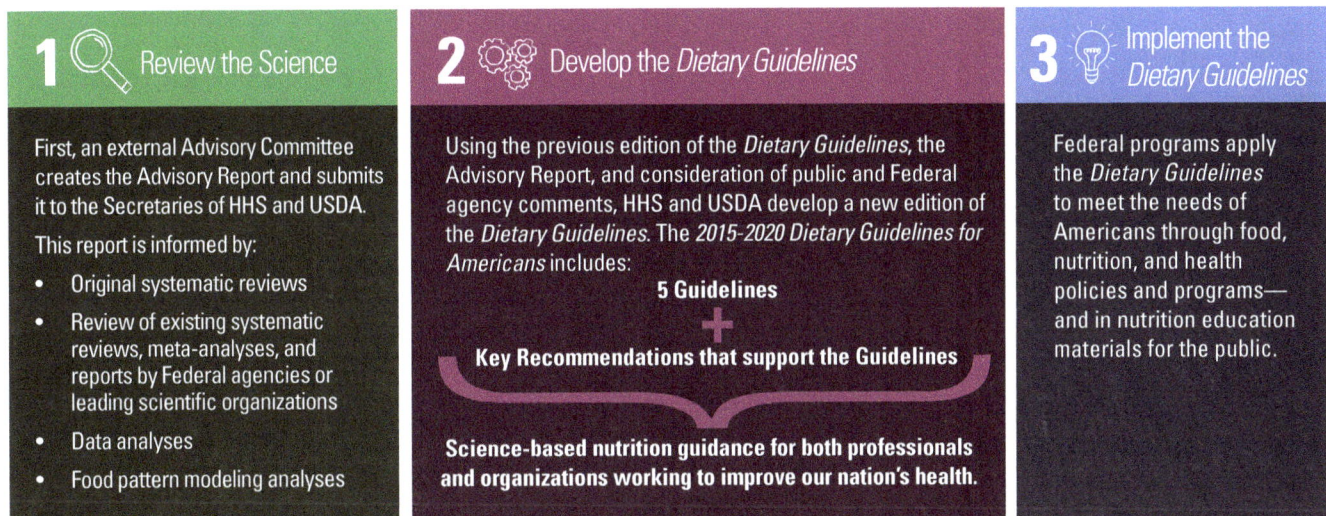

1 Review the Science	2 Develop the *Dietary Guidelines*	3 Implement the *Dietary Guidelines*
First, an external Advisory Committee creates the Advisory Report and submits it to the Secretaries of HHS and USDA. This report is informed by: • Original systematic reviews • Review of existing systematic reviews, meta-analyses, and reports by Federal agencies or leading scientific organizations • Data analyses • Food pattern modeling analyses	Using the previous edition of the *Dietary Guidelines*, the Advisory Report, and consideration of public and Federal agency comments, HHS and USDA develop a new edition of the *Dietary Guidelines*. The *2015-2020 Dietary Guidelines for Americans* includes: **5 Guidelines** **+** **Key Recommendations that support the Guidelines** **Science-based nutrition guidance for both professionals and organizations working to improve our nation's health.**	Federal programs apply the *Dietary Guidelines* to meet the needs of Americans through food, nutrition, and health policies and programs— and in nutrition education materials for the public.

[2] Public Law 101-445, Title III, Section 301, 7 U.S.C. 5341 et seq. requires that the U.S. Departments of Health and Human Services and of Agriculture publish a new edition of the *Dietary Guidelines for Americans* every 5 years.

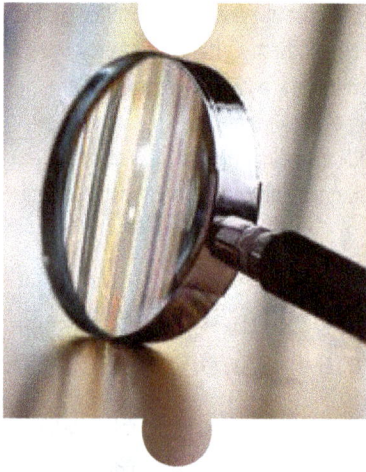

Stage 1: Review of Current Scientific Evidence

In the first stage, the Secretaries of HHS and of USDA appoint an external Dietary Guidelines Advisory Committee (Advisory Committee). The use of a Federal advisory committee is to ensure the Federal Government is seeking sound external scientific advice to inform policy decisions. Nominations from the public were sought for candidates to serve on the 2015 Advisory Committee. The 15 members of the 2015 Advisory Committee are prestigious researchers in the fields of nutrition, health, and medicine. Their role was to provide advice and recommendations to the Federal Government on the current state of scientific evidence on nutrition and health. Per Federal Advisory Committee Act rules, Advisory Committee members were thoroughly vetted for conflicts of interest before they were appointed to their positions and were required to submit a financial disclosure form annually.

The 2015 Advisory Committee was charged with reviewing the 2010 edition of the *Dietary Guidelines* to determine the topics for which new scientific evidence was likely to be available, and to review that evidence to inform the development of the 2015-2020 edition. The Advisory Committee was asked to place primary emphasis on evidence published since the 2010 Advisory Committee completed its work and on evidence to support the development of food-based recommendations that are of public health importance for Americans ages 2 years and older. It met in public meetings to discuss its findings and develop its recommendations. The public was invited to submit written comments to the Advisory Committee throughout the entirety of its work as well as oral comments at a public meeting.

The 2015 Advisory Committee used four state-of-the-art approaches to review and analyze the available evidence: original systematic reviews; existing systematic reviews, meta-analyses, and reports by Federal agencies or leading scientific organizations; data analyses; and food pattern modeling analyses. Most of its conclusion statements on nutrition and health were informed by systematic reviews, which are a gold standard for informing clinical practice guidelines and public health policies worldwide. The Dietary Reference Intakes (DRIs), as set by the Institute of Medicine (IOM), also serve as a source of evidence for the Advisory Report and the *Dietary Guidelines*. This multifaceted approach allowed the Advisory Committee to ask and answer scientific questions about the relationship of diet and health to systematically, objectively, and transparently synthesize research findings and to limit bias in its evaluation of the totality of the evidence for the topics it reviewed. This approach also allowed one or more methods to be used that were best suited to comprehensively answer each question. These methods are described here.

Original Systematic Reviews.

The Advisory Committee used this approach to systematically search the scientific literature for relevant articles; assess the methodologic rigor of each included article; and summarize, analyze, and grade the evidence presented in the articles.

For systematic reviews, all studies published by the time the literature search was conducted were screened for inclusion to ensure all available evidence was reviewed in a systematic manner. To preserve the integrity of the process, individual studies that were published after the systematic review was concluded were not included on an ad hoc basis. Recent studies that were not included in the 2015 Advisory Committee's review will be available for consideration during the development of the next edition of the *Dietary Guidelines*.

The USDA Nutrition Evidence Library (NEL) uses a systematic review methodology designed to analyze food, nutrition, and public health science. The medical field has used systematic reviews as the standard practice for more than 25 years to inform the development of national guidelines for health professionals.

Review of Existing Systematic Reviews, Meta-Analyses, and Reports by Federal Agencies or Leading Scientific Organizations.

The Advisory Committee used this method when a high-quality existing review or report had already addressed a question under consideration. The approach involved applying a systematic process to assess the quality of the existing review or report and to ensure that it presented a comprehensive review of the Advisory Committee's question of interest.

At the time that the NEL was created by USDA for use in informing the *2010 Dietary Guidelines*, it was among the first to apply the systematic review methodology in the field of nutrition. Thus, very few *existing* nutrition-focused systematic reviews were available for the 2010 Advisory Committee to use. Since that time, systematic reviews in the nutrition field have become common practice. Therefore, unlike the 2010 Advisory Committee, the 2015 Advisory Committee was able to use *existing* reviews to answer many of its research questions, preventing duplication of effort. Existing systematic reviews underwent quality assessment to ensure they were just as rigorous and were held to the same high standards as the systematic reviews conducted through the NEL.

Data Analyses. The Advisory Committee used national data from Federal agencies to answer questions about chronic disease prevalence rates; food and nutrient intakes of the U.S. population across age, sex, and other demographic characteristics; and nutrient content of foods.

For other questions, a new analysis from existing data sets was requested from the appropriate Federal agency to provide the answer to the question posed. Data analyses tailored to a specific question helped inform the Advisory Committee's recommendations.

Food Pattern Modeling Analyses. The Advisory Committee used this method to estimate the effect on diet quality of possible changes in types or amounts of foods in the USDA Food Patterns that it was considering recommending. The USDA Food Patterns describe the types and amounts of foods[3] to eat that can provide a healthy and nutritionally adequate diet. The Food Patterns aim to meet the DRIs while taking into consideration current intakes in the United States and systematic reviews of scientific research. They were developed to demonstrate how *Dietary Guidelines* recommendations can be met within an overall eating pattern.

Food pattern modeling analyses guided by the Advisory Committee provided objective information on the potential nutritional effects of recommending an eating pattern with specific changes, such as selecting foods to increase vitamin D intake or modifying the pattern based on studies of Mediterranean diets. The results of the modeling analyses informed the Committee's recommendations on specific topics, including keeping recommendations grounded within the structure of an overall healthy eating pattern.

As part of its assessment of evidence on diet and health, the Committee also formulated recommendations for future research. These research recommendations reflect an acknowledgment that knowledge about nutrition, diet, and health associations continues to evolve and that new findings build on and enhance existing evidence.

The Advisory Committee's work culminated in the *Scientific Report of the 2015 Dietary Guidelines Advisory Committee*, which was submitted to the Secretaries of HHS and of USDA and made available for public and agency comment in February 2015. For more information about the Advisory Committee and its review process and Advisory Report, visit http://health.gov/dietaryguidelines/.

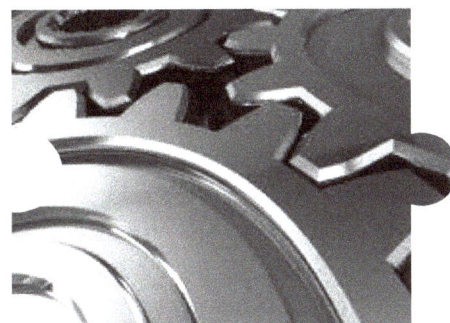

Stage 2: Development of the *Dietary Guidelines for Americans*

In the second stage, HHS and USDA develop the policy document *Dietary Guidelines*, applying several process steps to promote scientific rigor. Similar to previous editions, this 8th edition builds upon the preceding edition, with the scientific justification for revisions informed by the Advisory Committee's report and consideration of public and Federal agency comments.

As previously mentioned, the public is invited to submit written comments to the Advisory Committee throughout the entirety of its work as well as oral comments at a public meeting. In addition, after the Advisory Committee's report was submitted to the Secretaries, the public is again invited to submit written comments to the Federal Government on the Advisory Committee's final report as well as oral comments at a public meeting. Comments on the Advisory Committee's report are considered in the development of the policy document, placing emphasis on those with scientific justification while ensuring that the policy is based on the totality of the evidence and not on individual studies.

[3] If not specified explicitly, references to "foods" refer to "foods and beverages."

Federal agencies within HHS and USDA have extensive, broad scientific expertise in nutrition and health, as well as experts who specialize in unique aspects of nutrition and health. Federal experts validate the rigor of the policy document in multiple ways. After the Advisory Committee's report is complete, Federal agencies provide comments regarding the applicability and rigor of the report for consideration in translating the science into policy. Those who update the policy document are Federal experts with specialized knowledge in the evidence under consideration and its policy applications within the Federal Government. These policy writers include nutrition scientists,

Looking Ahead to 2020— Expanding Guidance

Traditionally, the *Dietary Guidelines* has focused on individuals ages 2 and older in the United States, including those who are at increased risk of chronic disease. This is the focus of the recommendations in this edition as well. However, the relationship of early nutrition to health outcomes throughout the lifespan has grown as a public health interest, and it is expected that evidence will become sufficiently robust to support additional dietary guidance in the future. As mandated by Congress in the Agricultural Act of 2014, also known as the Farm Bill, the *Dietary Guidelines* will expand to include infants and toddlers (from birth to age 2), as well as additional guidance for women who are pregnant, beginning with the 2020-2025 edition.

policy experts, and communications specialists. Consultation with other Federal experts occurs throughout the policy development process.

A peer-review step also is completed, in which nonfederal experts independently conduct a confidential review of the draft policy document for clarity and technical accuracy of the translation of the evidence from the Advisory Report into policy language. In addition, extensive review and clearance of the policy document also occurs by Federal experts within the agencies of both Departments. The Federal clearance of the policy document culminates with review and approval by the Secretaries of HHS and of USDA.

The *2015-2020 Dietary Guidelines* is built around five Guidelines with accompanying Key Recommendations that provide detail on the elements of healthy eating patterns. The Key Recommendations represent the preponderance of the most current scientific evidence. Emphasis is placed on topics with the strongest evidence or public health need, indicating a low likelihood that new or additional evidence would greatly change the recommendation. Ultimately, the *Dietary Guidelines* aims to represent the current science on diet and health, provide food-based guidance that meets nutrient needs, and address areas of particular public health importance in the United States.

Describing the Strength of Evidence Supporting Recommendations

Considerable evidence demonstrates that a healthy diet and regular physical activity can help improve health and reduce the risk of certain chronic diseases. Throughout, the 2015-2020 edition of the *Dietary Guidelines* notes the strength of evidence supporting its recommendations.

This information is provided to show how much evidence is available and how consistent the evidence is for a particular statement or recommendation:

Strong evidence reflects a large, high-quality, and/or consistent body of evidence. There is a high level of certainty that the evidence is relevant to the population of interest, and additional studies are unlikely to change conclusions derived from this evidence. Topics that are supported by strong evidence often lead to policy recommendations with the greatest emphasis because of the confidence generated by the evidence.

Moderate evidence reflects sufficient evidence to draw conclusions. The level of certainty may be restricted by certain limitations in the evidence, such as the amount of evidence available, inconsistencies in findings, or limitations in methodology or generalizability. Topics that are supported by moderate evidence can support recommendations of varying emphasis, including complementing those with a strong evidence base.

Limited evidence reflects either a small number of studies, studies of weak design or with inconsistent results, and/or limitations on the generalizability of the findings. When only limited evidence is available on a topic, it is insufficient to inform Key Recommendations. However, policy statements are sometimes useful for topics that have limited supporting evidence, such as when the evidence for those topics reinforces recommendations on related topics that have a stronger evidence base, to clarify that it is not possible to make a recommendation, or to identify an area of emerging research.

The evidence described in the *Dietary Guidelines* also reflects an understanding of the difference between *association* and *causation.* Two factors may be associated; however, this association does not mean that one factor necessarily causes the other. Often, several different factors may contribute to a health outcome. In some cases, scientific conclusions are based on relationships or associations because studies examining cause and effect are not available.

Stage 3: Implementing the *Dietary Guidelines for Americans*

In the third and final stage, the Federal Government implements the recommendations in the *Dietary Guidelines.* Federal programs apply the *Dietary Guidelines* to meet the needs of Americans and specific population groups through food, nutrition, and health policies and programs and in nutrition education materials for the public. Although the *Dietary Guidelines* provides the foundation for Federal nutrition and health initiatives, it is each Federal agency's purview and responsibility to determine how best to implement the *Dietary Guidelines* to serve its specific audiences. For example, one way USDA and other Federal agencies can implement the *Dietary Guidelines* is through MyPlate, which serves as a reminder to build healthy eating patterns by making healthy choices across the food groups. Both Federal and nonfederal programs may use MyPlate as a resource to help Americans make shifts in their daily food and beverage choices to align with the *Dietary Guidelines.* For more information about *Dietary Guidelines* implementation for the public through MyPlate, see Chapter 3. Everyone Has a Role To Play in Supporting Healthy Eating Patterns and Figure 3-2.

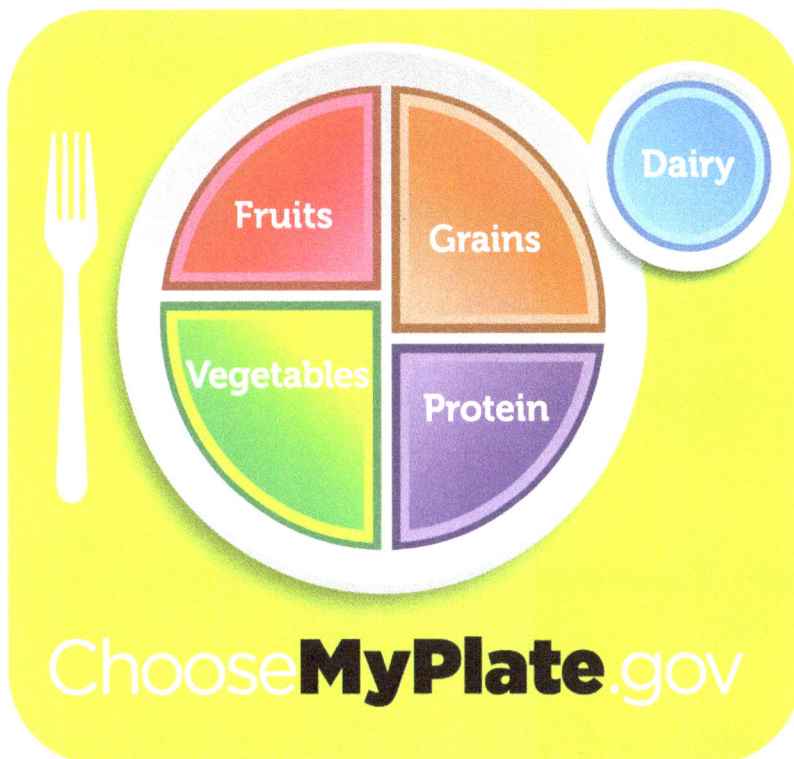

ChooseMyPlate.gov

Implementation of the *Dietary Guidelines* Through MyPlate

MyPlate is a Federal symbol that serves as a reminder to build healthy eating patterns by making healthy choices across the food groups. For more information about *Dietary Guidelines* implementation for the public through MyPlate, see Chapter 3 and **Figure 3-2.**

The *Dietary Guidelines* recognizes that many factors influence the diet and physical activity choices individuals make. The United States is a highly diverse nation, with people from many backgrounds, cultures, and traditions, and with varied personal preferences. It also acknowledges that income and life circumstances play a major role in food and physical activity decisions. Significant health and food access disparities exist, with nearly 15 percent of U.S. households unable to acquire adequate food to meet their needs because of insufficient income or other resources for food.[4] These factors—along with the settings in which people live, learn, work, and play—can have a profound impact on their choices.

In addition to implementation by the Federal Government and as discussed in Chapter 3, ample opportunities exist for many other sectors of society to implement the *Dietary Guidelines* in the multiple settings they influence, from home to school to work to community.

[4] U.S. Department of Agriculture. Economic Research Service. Food security in the U.S. Key Statistics and Graphics. [Updated September 8, 2015.] Available at: http://www.ers.usda.gov/topics/food-nutrition-assistance/food-security-in-the-us/key-statistics-graphics.aspx. Accessed June 10, 2015.

Aligning With the *Dietary Guidelines for Americans*: What Does This Mean in Practice?

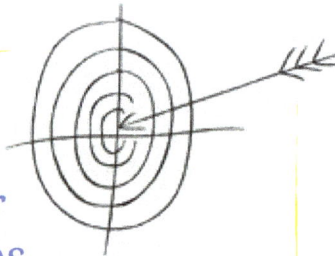

As introduced here and described in detail in the following Chapters, the *Dietary Guidelines* describes adaptable eating patterns that can help promote health and reduce risk of chronic disease across the lifespan. It presents an array of options that can be tailored to income levels and that can accommodate cultural, ethnic, traditional, and personal preferences.

All segments of society—individuals, families, communities, businesses and industries, organizations, governments, and others—can and should "align with the *Dietary Guidelines*." In practice, the goal is to take the following actions in their entirety and maintain them over time:

- Make food and beverage choices that meet the Key Recommendations for food groups, subgroups, nutrients, and other components in combination to contribute to overall healthy eating patterns.

- Meet nutritional needs primarily through foods. Foods provide an array of nutrients and other components that are associated with beneficial effects on health. Individuals should aim to consume a diet that achieves the most recent DRIs, which consider many factors, including the individual's age, life stage, and sex. In some cases, fortified foods and dietary supplements may be useful in providing one or more nutrients that otherwise may be consumed in less than recommended amounts or that are of particular concern for specific population groups.

- Establish and maintain settings (e.g., homes, schools, worksites, restaurants, stores) that support and encourage food and beverage choices that help individuals make shifts to meet the Key Recommendations for healthy eating patterns.

- Ensure that food is kept safe to eat by using the principles of clean, separate, cook, and chill.[5]

- Establish and maintain sectors and settings that support and encourage regular physical activity as part of a healthy lifestyle.

All of these actions are important individually, but they are intended to be taken together. Aligning with the *Dietary Guidelines* by taking these actions is powerful because it can help change social norms and values and ultimately support a new prevention and healthy lifestyle paradigm that will benefit the U.S. population today as well as future generations.

A Roadmap to the 2015-2020 Edition of the *Dietary Guidelines for Americans*

People do not eat foods and nutrients in isolation but in combination, and this combination forms an overall eating pattern. A growing body of research has examined the relationship between overall eating patterns, health, and risk of chronic disease, and findings on these relationships are sufficiently well established to support dietary guidance. As a result, eating patterns and their food and nutrient characteristics are a primary emphasis of the recommendations in this 2015-2020 edition of the *Dietary Guidelines*. This edition of the *Dietary Guidelines* consists of this Introduction, three chapters, and 14 appendixes:

- **Chapter 1. Key Elements of Healthy Eating Patterns** discusses the relationship of diet and physical activity to health over the lifespan and explains the principles of a healthy eating pattern. The chapter provides quantitative recommendations for a Healthy U.S.-Style Eating Pattern at the 2,000-calorie level as an example to show how individuals can follow these principles and recommendations. It also includes two variations at the same 2,000-calorie level as examples of other healthy eating patterns individuals can choose based on personal preference: the Healthy Mediterranean-Style Eating Pattern and the Healthy Vegetarian Eating Pattern. Chapter 1 focuses on the first three Guidelines and the Key Recommendations.

[5] For more information on this action, see Appendix 14. Food Safety Principles and Guidance.

- **Chapter 2. Shifts Needed To Align With Healthy Eating Patterns** compares current food and nutrient intakes in the United States to recommendations and describes the shifts in dietary choices that are needed to align current intakes with recommendations. Chapter 2 focuses on the fourth Guideline.

- **Chapter 3. Everyone Has a Role in Supporting Healthy Eating Patterns** explains how all individuals and segments of society in the United States have an important role to play in supporting healthy eating and physical activity choices. It outlines a variety of strategies and actions that align with the *Dietary Guidelines*. Chapter 3 focuses on the fifth Guideline.

- **The Appendixes** provide additional information to support the content of the chapters, including recommendations from the *Physical Activity Guidelines for Americans*; calorie needs by age, sex, and level of physical activity; the base Healthy U.S.-Style Eating Pattern; two other examples of healthy eating patterns: the Healthy Mediterranean-Style and Healthy Vegetarian Eating Patterns; a glossary of terms; and nutritional goals for various age-sex groups. The Appendixes also include a list of selected Government resources on diet and physical activity; additional information on alcohol; lists of food sources of nutrients of public health concern; and food safety principles and guidance.

Terms To Know

Several terms are used to operationalize the principles and recommendations of the *2015-2020 Dietary Guidelines*. These terms are essential to understanding the concepts discussed herein:

Eating Pattern—The combination of foods and beverages that constitute an individual's complete dietary intake over time. Often referred to as a "dietary pattern," an eating pattern may describe a customary way of eating or a combination of foods recommended for consumption. Specific examples include USDA Food Patterns and the Dietary Approaches to Stop Hypertension (DASH) Eating Plan.

Nutrient Dense—A characteristic of foods and beverages that provide vitamins, minerals, and other substances that contribute to adequate nutrient intakes or may have positive health effects, with little or no solid fats and added sugars, refined starches, and sodium. Ideally, these foods and beverages also are in forms that retain naturally occurring components, such as dietary fiber. All vegetables, fruits, whole grains, seafood, eggs, beans and peas, unsalted nuts and seeds, fat-free and low-fat dairy products, and lean meats and poultry—when prepared with little or no added solid fats, sugars, refined starches, and sodium—are nutrient-dense foods. These foods contribute to meeting food group recommendations within calorie and sodium limits. The term "nutrient dense" indicates the nutrients and other beneficial substances in a food have not been "diluted" by the addition of calories from added solid fats, sugars, or refined starches, or by the solid fats naturally present in the food.

Variety—A diverse assortment of foods and beverages across and within all food groups and subgroups selected to fulfill the recommended amounts without exceeding the limits for calories and other dietary components. For example, in the vegetables food group, selecting a variety of foods could be accomplished over the course of a week by choosing from all subgroups, including dark green, red and orange, legumes (beans and peas), starchy, and other vegetables.

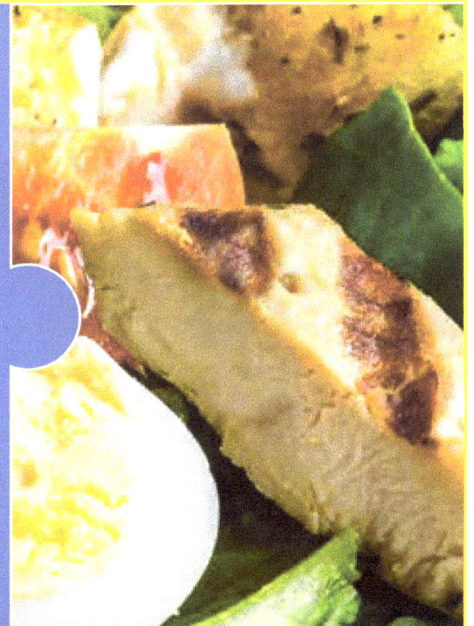

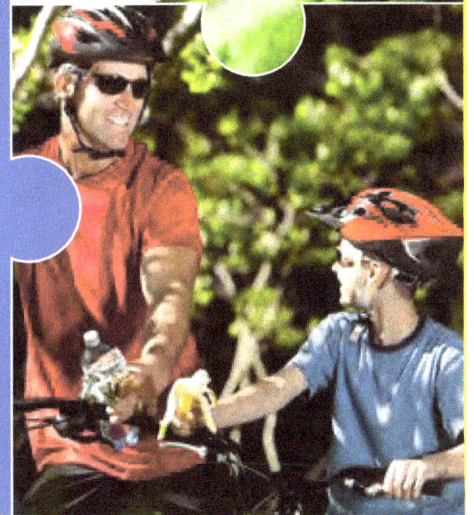

Key Elements of Healthy Eating Patterns

Introduction

Over the course of any given day, week, or year, individuals consume foods and beverages[1] in combination—an eating pattern. An eating pattern is more than the sum of its parts; it represents the totality of what individuals habitually eat and drink, and these dietary components act synergistically in relation to health. As a result, the eating pattern may be more predictive of overall health status and disease risk than individual foods or nutrients. Thus, eating patterns, and their food and nutrient components, are at the core of the *2015-2020 Dietary Guidelines for Americans*. The goal of the *Dietary Guidelines* is for individuals throughout all stages of the lifespan to have eating patterns that promote overall health and help prevent chronic disease.

About This Chapter

This chapter defines the core concepts of healthy eating and physical activity patterns and focuses on the first three Guidelines:

1. **Follow a healthy eating pattern across the lifespan.** All food and beverage choices matter. Choose a healthy eating pattern at an appropriate calorie level to help achieve and maintain a healthy body weight, support nutrient adequacy, and reduce the risk of chronic disease.

2. **Focus on variety, nutrient density, and amount.** To meet nutrient needs within calorie limits, choose a variety of nutrient-dense foods across and within all food groups in recommended amounts.

3. **Limit calories from added sugars and saturated fats and reduce sodium intake.** Consume an eating pattern low in added sugars, saturated fats, and sodium. Cut back on foods and beverages higher in these components to amounts that fit within healthy eating patterns.

4. **Shift to healthier food and beverage choices.** Choose nutrient-dense foods and beverages across and within all food groups in place of less healthy choices. Consider cultural and personal preferences to make these shifts easier to accomplish and maintain.

5. **Support healthy eating patterns for all.** Everyone has a role in helping to create and support healthy eating patterns in multiple settings nationwide, from home to school to work to communities.

The chapter first presents Key Recommendations, which describe the elements of a healthy eating pattern and provide detail on how individuals can follow the Guidelines, followed by a description of the science supporting healthy eating patterns. Then, the Healthy U.S.-Style Eating Pattern at the 2,000-calorie level is provided as an example. A Closer Look Inside a Healthy Eating Pattern provides details on each of the food groups and other dietary components of public health importance in the United States. In addition, the chapter provides two variations of the Healthy U.S.-Style Eating Pattern as examples of additional healthy eating patterns—the Healthy Mediterranean-Style Eating Pattern and the Healthy Vegetarian Eating Pattern. Both of these patterns align with the Guidelines. Finally, this chapter provides an overview of healthy physical activity patterns.

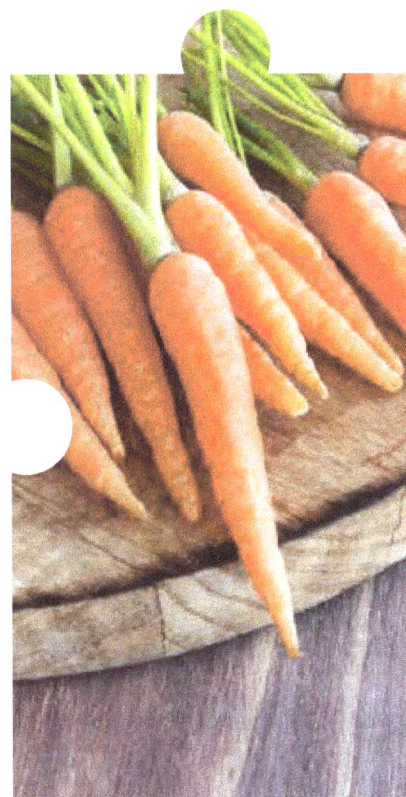

[1] If not specified explicitly, references to "foods" refer to "foods and beverages."

Key Recommendations: Components of Healthy Eating Patterns

The *Dietary Guidelines'* Key Recommendations for healthy eating patterns should be applied in their entirety, given the interconnected relationship that each dietary component can have with others. As illustrated later in this chapter, there is more than one way to put these Key Recommendations into action; this is exemplified by the three eating patterns that translate and integrate the Key Recommendations into an overall healthy way to eat.

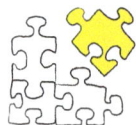

Key Recommendations:

Consume a healthy eating pattern that accounts for all foods and beverages within an appropriate calorie level.

A healthy eating pattern includes:[2]

- A variety of vegetables from all of the subgroups—dark green, red and orange, legumes (beans and peas), starchy, and other
- Fruits, especially whole fruits
- Grains, at least half of which are whole grains
- Fat-free or low-fat dairy, including milk, yogurt, cheese, and/or fortified soy beverages
- A variety of protein foods, including seafood, lean meats and poultry, eggs, legumes (beans and peas), and nuts, seeds, and soy products
- Oils

A healthy eating pattern limits:

- Saturated fats and *trans* fats, added sugars, and sodium

Key Recommendations that are quantitative are provided for several components of the diet that should be limited. These components are of particular public health concern in the United States, and the specified limits can help individuals achieve healthy eating patterns within calorie limits:

- Consume less than 10 percent of calories per day from added sugars[3]
- Consume less than 10 percent of calories per day from saturated fats[4]
- Consume less than 2,300 milligrams (mg) per day of sodium[5]
- If alcohol is consumed, it should be consumed in moderation—up to one drink per day for women and up to two drinks per day for men—and only by adults of legal drinking age.[6]

[2] Definitions for each food group and subgroup are provided throughout the chapter and are compiled in Appendix 3. USDA Food Patterns: Healthy U.S.-Style Eating Pattern.

[3] The recommendation to limit intake of calories from added sugars to less than 10 percent per day is a target based on food pattern modeling and national data on intakes of calories from added sugars that demonstrate the public health need to limit calories from added sugars to meet food group and nutrient needs within calorie limits. The limit on calories from added sugars is not a Tolerable Upper Intake Level (UL) set by the Institute of Medicine (IOM). For most calorie levels, there are not enough calories available after meeting food group needs to consume 10 percent of calories from added sugars and 10 percent of calories from saturated fats and still stay within calorie limits.

[4] The recommendation to limit intake of calories from saturated fats to less than 10 percent per day is a target based on evidence that replacing saturated fats with unsaturated fats is associated with reduced risk of cardiovascular disease. The limit on calories from saturated fats is not a UL set by the IOM. For most calorie levels, there are not enough calories available after meeting food group needs to consume 10 percent of calories from added sugars and 10 percent of calories from saturated fats and still stay within calorie limits.

[5] The recommendation to limit intake of sodium to less than 2,300 mg per day is the UL for individuals ages 14 years and older set by the IOM. The recommendations for children younger than 14 years of age are the IOM age- and sex-appropriate ULs (see Appendix 7. Nutritional Goals for Age-Sex Groups Based on Dietary Reference Intakes and Dietary Guidelines Recommendations).

[6] It is not recommended that individuals begin drinking or drink more for any reason. The amount of alcohol and calories in beverages varies and should be accounted for within the limits of healthy eating patterns. Alcohol should be consumed only by adults of legal drinking age. There are many circumstances in which individuals should not drink, such as during pregnancy. See Appendix 9. Alcohol for additional information.

Healthy Eating Patterns: Dietary Principles

Healthy eating patterns support a healthy body weight and can help prevent and reduce the risk of chronic disease throughout periods of growth, development, and aging as well as during pregnancy. The following principles apply to meeting the Key Recommendations:

An eating pattern represents the totality of all foods and beverages consumed. All foods consumed as part of a healthy eating pattern fit together like a puzzle to meet nutritional needs without exceeding limits, such as those for saturated fats, added sugars, sodium, and total calories. All forms of foods, including fresh, canned, dried, and frozen, can be included in healthy eating patterns.

Nutritional needs should be met primarily from foods. Individuals should aim to meet their nutrient needs through healthy eating patterns that include nutrient-dense foods. Foods in nutrient-dense forms contain essential vitamins and minerals and also dietary fiber and other naturally occurring substances that may have positive health effects. In some cases, fortified foods and dietary supplements may be useful in providing one or more nutrients that otherwise may be consumed in less than recommended amounts (see Chapter 2. Shifts Needed To Align With Healthy Eating Patterns).

Healthy eating patterns are adaptable. Individuals have more than one way to achieve a healthy eating pattern. Any eating pattern can be tailored to the individual's socio-cultural and personal preferences.

Healthy Physical Activity Patterns

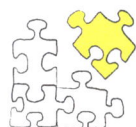

Key Recommendation:

Meet the *Physical Activity Guidelines for Americans*

In addition to consuming a healthy eating pattern, individuals in the United States should meet the *Physical Activity Guidelines for Americans*.[7] Regular physical activity is one of the most important things individuals can do to improve their health. The *Physical Activity Guidelines*, released by the U.S. Department of Health and Human Services, provides a comprehensive set of recommendations for Americans on the amounts and types of physical activity needed each day (see Appendix 1. *Physical Activity Guidelines for Americans*). Adults need at least 150 minutes of moderate intensity physical activity and should perform muscle-strengthening exercises on 2 or more days each week. Youth ages 6 to 17 years need at least 60 minutes of physical activity per day, including aerobic, muscle-strengthening, and bone-strengthening activities. Establishing and maintaining a regular physical activity pattern can provide many health benefits. Strong evidence shows that regular physical activity helps people maintain a healthy weight, prevent excessive weight gain, and lose weight when combined with a healthy eating pattern lower in calories. Strong evidence also demonstrates that regular physical activity lowers the risk of early death, coronary heart disease, stroke, high blood pressure, adverse blood lipid profile, type 2 diabetes, breast and colon cancer, and metabolic syndrome; it also reduces depression and prevents falls. People can engage in regular physical activity in a variety of ways throughout the day and by choosing activities they enjoy. The *Physical Activity Guidelines* provides additional details on the benefits of physical activity and strategies to incorporate regular physical activity into a healthy lifestyle.

[7] U.S. Department of Health and Human Services. 2008 *Physical Activity Guidelines for Americans.* Washington (DC): U.S. Department of Health and Human Services; 2008. ODPHP Publication No. U0036. Available at: http://www.health.gov/paguidelines. Accessed August 6, 2015.

The Science Behind Healthy Eating Patterns

The components of healthy eating patterns recommended in this edition of the *Dietary Guidelines* were developed by integrating findings from systematic reviews of scientific research, food pattern modeling, and analyses of current intake of the U.S. population:

- Systematic reviews of scientific research examine relationships between the overall diet, including its constituent foods, beverages, and nutrients, and health outcomes.

- Food pattern modeling assesses how well various combinations and amounts of foods from all food groups would result in healthy eating patterns that meet nutrient needs and accommodate limits, such as those for saturated fats, added sugars, and sodium.

- Analyses of current intakes identify areas of potential public health concern.

Together, these complementary approaches provide a robust evidence base for healthy eating patterns that both reduce risk of diet-related chronic disease and ensure nutrient adequacy.

Scientific evidence supporting dietary guidance has grown and evolved over the decades. Previous editions of the *Dietary Guidelines* relied on the evidence of relationships between individual nutrients, foods, and food groups and health outcomes. Although this evidence base continues to be substantial, foods are not consumed in isolation, but rather in various combinations over time—an "eating pattern." As previously noted, dietary components of an eating pattern can have interactive, synergistic, and potentially cumulative relationships, such that the eating pattern may be more predictive of overall health status and disease risk than individual foods or nutrients. However, each identified component of an eating pattern does not necessarily have the same independent relationship to health outcomes as the total eating pattern, and each identified component may not equally contribute (or may be a marker for other factors) to the associated health outcome. An evidence base is now available that evaluates overall eating patterns and various health outcomes.

Associations Between Eating Patterns & Health

Evidence shows that healthy eating patterns, as outlined in the Guidelines and Key Recommendations, are associated with positive health outcomes. The evidence base for associations between eating patterns and specific health outcomes continues to grow. Strong evidence shows that healthy eating patterns are associated with a reduced risk of cardiovascular disease (CVD). Moderate evidence indicates that healthy eating patterns also are associated with a reduced risk of type 2 diabetes, certain types of cancers (such as colorectal and postmenopausal breast cancers), overweight, and obesity. Emerging evidence also suggests that relationships may exist between eating patterns and some neurocognitive disorders and congenital anomalies.

Within this body of evidence, higher intakes of vegetables and fruits consistently have been identified as characteristics of healthy eating patterns; whole grains have been identified as well, although with slightly less consistency. Other characteristics of healthy eating patterns have been identified with less consistency and include fat-free or low-fat dairy, seafood, legumes, and nuts. Lower intakes of meats, including processed meats; processed poultry; sugar-sweetened foods, particularly beverages; and refined grains have often been identified as characteristics of healthy eating patterns. Additional information about how food groups and dietary components fit within healthy eating patterns is discussed throughout the *2015-2020 Dietary Guidelines*. For example, as discussed later in this chapter in the section About Meats and Poultry, evidence from food pattern modeling has demonstrated that lean meats can be part of a healthy eating pattern, but as discussed in Chapter 2, average intakes of meats, poultry, and eggs, a subgroup of the protein foods group, are above recommendations in the Healthy U.S.-Style Eating Pattern for teen boys and adult men.

Associations Between Dietary Components & Health

The evidence on food groups and various health outcomes that is reflected in this 2015-2020 edition of the *Dietary Guidelines* complements and builds on the evidence of the previous 2010 edition. For example, research has shown that vegetables and fruits are associated with a reduced risk of many chronic diseases, including CVD, and may be protective against certain types of cancers. Additionally, some evidence indicates that whole grain intake may reduce risk for CVD and is associated with lower body weight. Research also has linked dairy intake to improved bone health, especially in children and adolescents.

A Closer Look Inside Healthy Eating Patterns

The following sections describe a healthy eating pattern and how following such a pattern can help people meet the Guidelines and its Key Recommendations. Throughout, it uses the Healthy U.S.-Style Eating Pattern as an example to illustrate the specific amounts and limits for food groups and other dietary components that make up healthy eating patterns. The Healthy U.S.-Style Eating Pattern is one of three USDA Food Patterns and is based on the types and proportions of foods Americans typically consume, but in nutrient-dense forms and appropriate amounts. Because calorie needs vary based on age, sex, height, weight, and level of physical activity (see Appendix 2. Estimated Calorie Needs per Day, by Age, Sex, and Physical Activity Level), the pattern has been provided at 12 different calorie levels (see Appendix 3. USDA Food Patterns: Healthy U.S.-Style Eating Pattern). The 2,000-calorie level of the Pattern is shown in **Table 1-1**.

The Healthy U.S.-Style Eating Pattern is the same as the primary USDA Food Patterns of the *2010 Dietary Guidelines*. Two additional USDA Food Patterns—the Healthy Mediterranean-Style Eating Pattern and the Healthy Vegetarian Eating Pattern—are found at the end of this chapter and reflect other styles of eating (see Appendix 4. USDA Food Patterns: Healthy Mediterranean-Style Eating Pattern and Appendix 5. USDA Food Patterns: Healthy Vegetarian Eating Pattern). These three patterns are examples of healthy eating patterns that can be adapted based on cultural and personal preferences. The USDA Food Patterns also can be used as guides to plan and serve meals not only for the individual and household but in a variety of other settings, including schools, worksites, and other community settings.

Table 1-1.

Healthy U.S.-Style Eating Pattern at the 2,000-Calorie Level, With Daily or Weekly Amounts From Food Groups, Subgroups, & Components

Food Group[a]	Amount[b] in the 2,000-Calorie-Level Pattern
Vegetables	**2½ c-eq/day**
Dark Green	1½ c-eq/wk
Red & Orange	5½ c-eq/wk
Legumes (Beans & Peas)	1½ c-eq/wk
Starchy	5 c-eq/wk
Other	4 c-eq/wk
Fruits	**2 c-eq/day**
Grains	**6 oz-eq/day**
Whole Grains	≥ 3 oz-eq/day
Refined Grains	≤ 3 oz-eq/day
Dairy	**3 c-eq/day**
Protein Foods	**5½ oz-eq/day**
Seafood	8 oz-eq/wk
Meats, Poultry, Eggs	26 oz-eq/wk
Nuts, Seeds, Soy Products	5 oz-eq/wk
Oils	**27 g/day**
Limit on Calories for Other Uses (% of Calories)[c]	**270 kcal/day (14%)**

[a] Definitions for each food group and subgroup are provided throughout the chapter and are compiled in Appendix 3.

[b] Food group amounts shown in cup-(c) or ounce-(oz) equivalents (eq). Oils are shown in grams (g). Quantity equivalents for each food group are defined in Appendix 3. Amounts will vary for those who need less than 2,000 or more than 2,000 calories per day. See Appendix 3 for all 12 calorie levels of the pattern.

[c] Assumes food choices to meet food group recommendations are in nutrient-dense forms. Calories from added sugars, added refined starches, solid fats, alcohol, and/or to eat more than the recommended amount of nutrient-dense foods are accounted for under this category.

NOTE: The total eating pattern should not exceed *Dietary Guidelines* limits for intake of calories from added sugars and saturated fats and alcohol and should be within the Acceptable Macronutrient Distribution Ranges for calories from protein, carbohydrate, and total fats. Most calorie patterns do not have enough calories available after meeting food group needs to consume 10 percent of calories from added sugars and 10 percent of calories from saturated fats and still stay within calorie limits. Values are rounded.

The Healthy U.S.-Style Eating Pattern is designed to meet the Recommended Dietary Allowances (RDA) and Adequate Intakes for essential nutrients, as well as Acceptable Macronutrient Distribution Ranges (AMDR) set by the Food and Nutrition Board of the IOM. This eating pattern also conforms to limits set by the IOM or *Dietary Guidelines* for other nutrients or food components (see Appendix 6. Glossary of Terms and Appendix 7. Nutritional Goals for Age-Sex Groups Based on Dietary Reference Intakes and Dietary Guidelines Recommendations). Nutritional goals for almost all nutrients are met (see Appendix 3 for additional information).

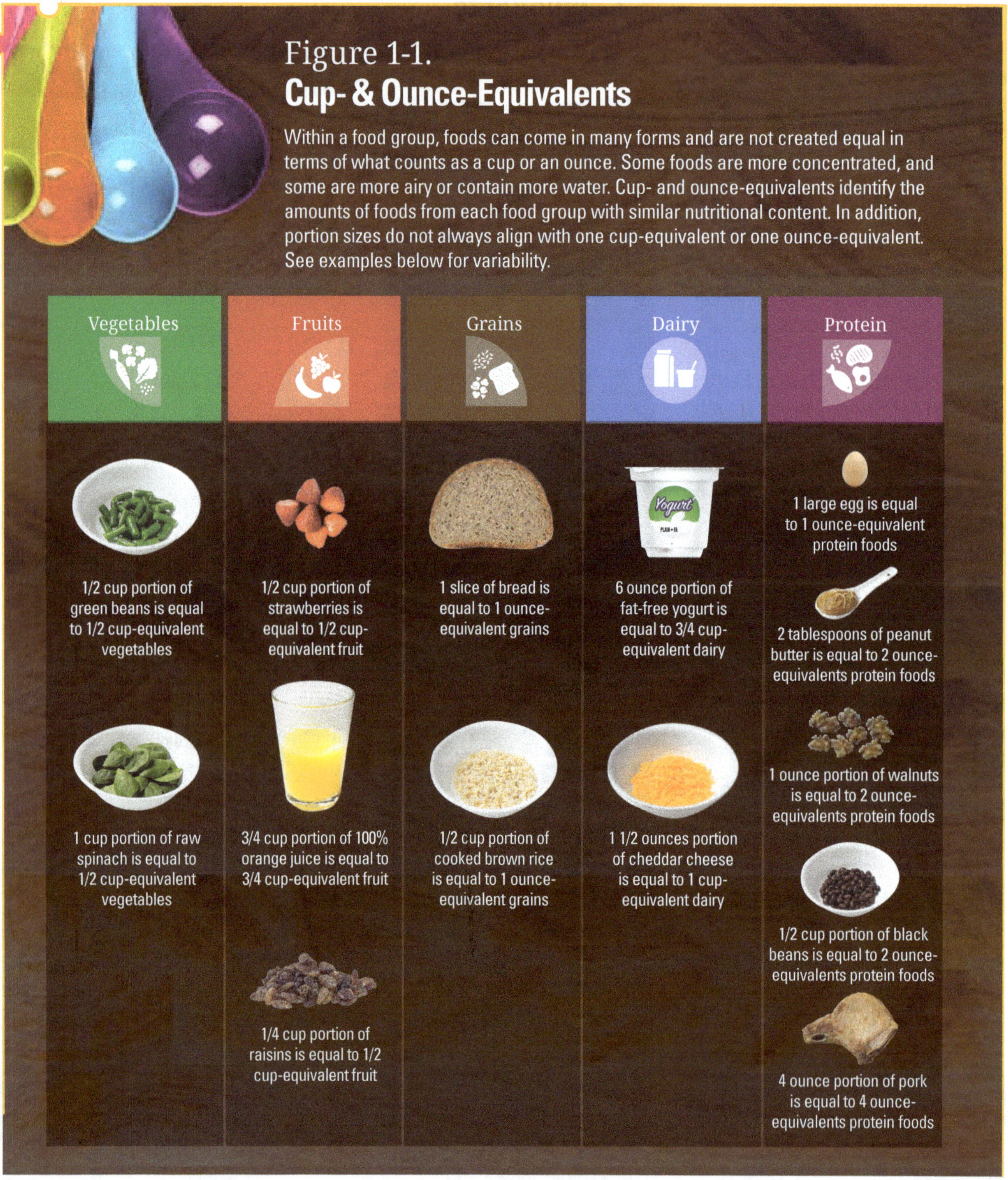

Figure 1-1.
Cup- & Ounce-Equivalents

Within a food group, foods can come in many forms and are not created equal in terms of what counts as a cup or an ounce. Some foods are more concentrated, and some are more airy or contain more water. Cup- and ounce-equivalents identify the amounts of foods from each food group with similar nutritional content. In addition, portion sizes do not always align with one cup-equivalent or one ounce-equivalent. See examples below for variability.

Vegetables	Fruits	Grains	Dairy	Protein
1/2 cup portion of green beans is equal to 1/2 cup-equivalent vegetables	1/2 cup portion of strawberries is equal to 1/2 cup-equivalent fruit	1 slice of bread is equal to 1 ounce-equivalent grains	6 ounce portion of fat-free yogurt is equal to 3/4 cup-equivalent dairy	1 large egg is equal to 1 ounce-equivalent protein foods
1 cup portion of raw spinach is equal to 1/2 cup-equivalent vegetables	3/4 cup portion of 100% orange juice is equal to 3/4 cup-equivalent fruit	1/2 cup portion of cooked brown rice is equal to 1 ounce-equivalent grains	1 1/2 ounces portion of cheddar cheese is equal to 1 cup-equivalent dairy	2 tablespoons of peanut butter is equal to 2 ounce-equivalents protein foods
	1/4 cup portion of raisins is equal to 1/2 cup-equivalent fruit			1 ounce portion of walnuts is equal to 2 ounce-equivalents protein foods
				1/2 cup portion of black beans is equal to 2 ounce-equivalents protein foods
				4 ounce portion of pork is equal to 4 ounce-equivalents protein foods

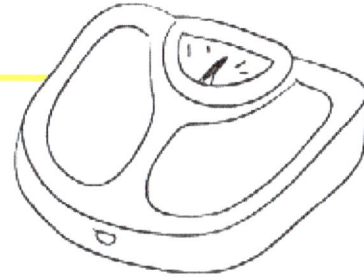

Importance of Calorie Balance Within Healthy Eating Patterns

Managing calorie intake is fundamental to achieving and maintaining calorie balance—the balance between the calories taken in from foods and the calories expended from metabolic processes and physical activity. The best way to determine whether an eating pattern is at an appropriate number of calories is to monitor body weight and adjust calorie intake and expenditure in physical activity based on changes in weight over time.

All foods and many beverages contain calories, and the total number of calories varies depending on the macronutrients in a food. On average, carbohydrates and protein contain 4 calories per gram, fats contain 9 calories per gram, and alcohol has 7 calories per gram. The total number of calories a person needs each day varies depending on a number of factors, including the person's age, sex, height, weight, and level of physical activity (see Appendix 2). In addition, a need to lose, maintain, or gain weight and other factors affect how many calories should be consumed.

All Americans—children, adolescents, adults, and older adults—are encouraged to achieve and/or maintain a healthy body weight. General guidance for achieving and maintaining a healthy body weight is provided below, and Appendix 8. Federal Resources for Information on Nutrition and Physical Activity provides additional resources, including an evolving array of tools to facilitate Americans' adoption of healthy choices.

- Children and adolescents are encouraged to maintain calorie balance to support normal growth and development without promoting excess weight gain. Children and adolescents who are overweight or obese should change their eating and physical activity behaviors to maintain or reduce their rate of weight gain while linear growth occurs, so that they can reduce body mass index (BMI) percentile toward a healthy range.

- Before becoming pregnant, women are encouraged to achieve and maintain a healthy weight, and women who are pregnant are encouraged to gain weight within gestational weight gain guidelines.[8]

- Adults who are obese should change their eating and physical activity behaviors to prevent additional weight gain and/or promote weight loss. Adults who are overweight should not gain additional weight, and those with one or more CVD risk factors (e.g., hypertension and hyperlipidemia) should change their eating and physical activity behaviors to lose weight. To lose weight, most people need to reduce the number of calories they get from foods and beverages and increase their physical activity. For a weight loss of 1 to 1½ pounds per week, daily intake should be reduced by 500 to 750 calories. Eating patterns that contain 1,200 to 1,500 calories each day can help most women lose weight safely, and eating patterns that contain 1,500 to 1,800 calories each day are suitable for most men for weight loss. In adults who are overweight or obese, if reduction in total calorie intake is achieved, a variety of eating patterns can produce weight loss, particularly in the first 6 months to 2 years;[9] however, more research is needed on the health implications of consuming these eating patterns long-term.

- Older adults, ages 65 years and older, who are overweight or obese are encouraged to prevent additional weight gain. Among older adults who are obese, particularly those with CVD risk factors, intentional weight loss can be beneficial and result in improved quality of life and reduced risk of chronic diseases and associated disabilities.

[8] Institute of Medicine (IOM) and National Research Council (NRC). Weight gain during pregnancy: Reexamining the guidelines. Washington (DC): The National Academies Press; 2009.

[9] Jensen MD, Ryan DH, Apovian CM, Ard JD, Comuzzie AG, Donato KA, et al. 2013 AHA/ACC/TOS guideline for the management of overweight and obesity in adults: a report of the American College of Cardiology/American Heart Association Task Force on Practice Guidelines and The Obesity Society. J Am Coll Cardiol. 2014;63(25 Pt B):2985-3023. PMID: 24239920. Available at: http://www.ncbi.nlm.nih.gov/pubmed/24239920.

Food Groups

Eating an appropriate mix of foods from the food groups and subgroups—within an appropriate calorie level—is important to promote health. Each of the food groups and their subgroups provides an array of nutrients, and the amounts recommended reflect eating patterns that have been associated with positive health outcomes. Foods from all of the food groups should be eaten in nutrient-dense forms. The following sections describe the recommendations for each of the food groups, highlight nutrients for which the food group is a key contributor, and describe special considerations related to the food group.

Vegetables

Healthy Intake: Healthy eating patterns include a variety of vegetables from all of the five vegetable subgroups—dark green, red and orange, legumes (beans and peas), starchy, and other.[10] These include all fresh, frozen, canned, and dried options in cooked or raw forms, including vegetable juices. The recommended amount of vegetables in the Healthy U.S.-Style Eating Pattern at the 2,000-calorie level is 2½ cup-equivalents of vegetables per day. In addition, weekly amounts from each vegetable subgroup are recommended to ensure variety and meet nutrient needs.

Key Nutrient Contributions: Vegetables are important sources of many nutrients, including dietary fiber, potassium, vitamin A,[11] vitamin C, vitamin K, copper, magnesium, vitamin E, vitamin B6, folate, iron, manganese, thiamin, niacin, and choline. Each of the vegetable subgroups contributes different combinations of nutrients, making it important for individuals to consume vegetables from all the subgroups. For example, dark-green vegetables provide the most vitamin K, red

About Legumes (Beans & Peas)

Legumes include kidney beans, pinto beans, white beans, black beans, garbanzo beans (chickpeas), lima beans (mature, dried), split peas, lentils, and edamame (green soybeans).

Legumes are excellent sources of protein. In addition, they provide other nutrients that also are found in seafood, meats, and poultry, such as iron and zinc. They are excellent sources of dietary fiber and of nutrients, such as potassium and folate that also are found in other vegetables.

Because legumes have a similar nutrient profile to foods in both the protein foods group and the vegetable group, they may be thought of as either a vegetable or a protein food and thus, can be counted as a vegetable or a protein food to meet recommended intakes.

Green peas and green (string) beans are not counted in the legume subgroup, because their nutrient compositions are not similar to legumes. Green peas are similar to starchy vegetables and are grouped with them. Green beans are grouped with the other vegetables subgroup, which includes onions, iceberg lettuce, celery, and cabbage, because their nutrient content is not similar to legumes.

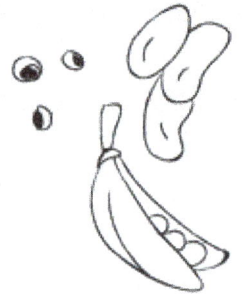

and orange vegetables the most vitamin A, legumes the most dietary fiber, and starchy vegetables the most potassium. Vegetables in the "other" vegetable subgroup provide a wide range of nutrients in varying amounts.

Considerations: To provide all of the nutrients and potential health benefits that vary across different types of vegetables, the Healthy U.S.-Style Eating Pattern includes weekly recommendations for each subgroup. Vegetable choices over time should vary and include many different vegetables. Vegetables should be consumed in a nutrient-dense form, with limited additions such as salt, butter, or creamy sauces. When selecting frozen or canned vegetables, choose those lower in sodium.

Fruits

Healthy Intake: Healthy eating patterns include fruits, especially whole fruits. The fruits food group includes whole fruits

and 100% fruit juice. Whole fruits include fresh, canned, frozen, and dried forms. The recommended amount of fruits in the Healthy U.S.-Style Eating Pattern at the 2,000-calorie level is 2 cup-equivalents per day. One cup of 100% fruit juice counts as 1 cup of fruit. Although fruit juice can be part of healthy eating patterns, it is lower than whole fruit in dietary fiber and when consumed in excess can contribute extra calories. Therefore, at least half of the recommended amount of fruits should come from whole fruits. When juices are consumed, they should be 100% juice, without added sugars. Also, when selecting canned fruit, choose options that are lowest in added sugars. One-half cup of dried fruit counts as one cup-equivalent of fruit. Similar to juice, when consumed in excess, dried fruits can contribute extra calories.

Key Nutrient Contributions: Among the many nutrients fruits provide are dietary fiber, potassium, and vitamin C.

[10] Definitions for each food group and subgroup are provided throughout the chapter and are compiled in Appendix 3.

[11] In the form of provitamin A carotenoids

Considerations: Juices may be partially fruit juice, and only the proportion that is 100% fruit juice counts (e.g., 1 cup of juice that is 50% juice counts as ½ cup of fruit juice). The remainder of the product may contain added sugars. Sweetened juice products with minimal juice content, such as juice drinks, are considered to be sugar-sweetened beverages rather than fruit juice because they are primarily composed of water with added sugars (see the Added Sugars section). The percent of juice in a beverage may be found on the package label, such as "contains 25% juice" or "100% fruit juice." The amounts of fruit juice allowed in the USDA Food Patterns for young children align with the recommendation from the American Academy of Pediatrics that young children consume no more than 4 to 6 fluid ounces of 100% fruit juice per day.[12] Fruits with small amounts of added sugars can be accommodated in the diet as long as calories from added sugars do not exceed 10 percent per day and total calorie intake remains within limits.

Grains

Healthy Intake: Healthy eating patterns include whole grains and limit the intake of refined grains and products made with refined grains, especially those high in saturated fats, added sugars, and/or sodium, such as cookies, cakes, and some snack foods. The grains food group includes grains as single foods (e.g., rice, oatmeal, and popcorn), as well as products that include grains as an ingredient (e.g., breads, cereals, crackers, and pasta). Grains are either whole or refined. Whole grains (e.g., brown rice, quinoa, and oats) contain the entire kernel, including the endosperm, bran, and germ. Refined grains differ from whole grains

in that the grains have been processed to remove the bran and germ, which removes dietary fiber, iron, and other nutrients. The recommended amount of grains in the Healthy U.S.-Style Eating Pattern at the 2,000-calorie level is 6 ounce-equivalents per day. At least half of this amount should be whole grains (see the How To Make at Least Half of Grains Whole Grains call-out box).

Key Nutrient Contributions: Whole grains are a source of nutrients, such as dietary fiber, iron, zinc, manganese, folate, magnesium, copper, thiamin, niacin, vitamin B6, phosphorus, selenium, riboflavin, and vitamin A.[13] Whole grains vary in their dietary fiber content. Most refined grains are enriched, a process that adds back iron and four B vitamins (thiamin, riboflavin, niacin, and folic acid). Because of this process, the term "enriched grains" is often used to describe these refined grains.

Considerations: Individuals who eat refined grains should choose enriched grains. Those who consume all of their grains as whole grains should include some grains, such as some whole-grain ready-to-eat breakfast cereals, that have been fortified with folic acid. This is particularly important for women who are or are capable of becoming pregnant, as folic acid fortification in the United States has been successful in reducing the incidence of neural tube defects during fetal development. Although grain products that are high in added sugars and saturated fats, such as cookies, cakes, and some snack foods, should be limited, as discussed in the Added Sugars and Saturated Fats sections, grains with some added sugars and saturated fats can fit within healthy eating patterns.

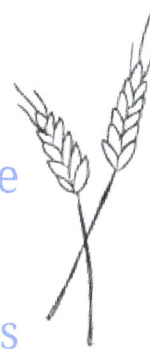

How To Make at Least Half of Grains Whole Grains

A food is a 100-percent whole-grain food if the only grains it contains are whole grains. One ounce-equivalent of whole grains has 16 g of whole grains. The recommendation to consume at least half of total grains as whole grains can be met in a number of ways.

The most direct way to meet the whole grain recommendation is to choose 100 percent whole-grain foods for at least half of all grains consumed. The relative amount of whole grain in the food can be inferred by the placement of the grain in the ingredients list. The whole grain should be the first ingredient—or the second ingredient, after water. For foods with multiple whole-grain ingredients, they should appear near the beginning of the ingredients list.

Many grain foods contain both whole grains and refined grains. These foods also can help people meet the whole grain recommendation, especially if a considerable proportion of the grain ingredients is whole grains. Another way to meet the recommendation to make at least half of grains whole grains is to choose products with at least 50 percent of the total weight as whole-grain ingredients.[14],[15] If a food has at least 8 g of whole grains per ounce-equivalent, it is at least half whole grains.[16] Some product labels show the whole grains health claim or the grams of whole grain in the product. This information may help people identify food choices that have a substantial amount of whole grains.

[12] American Academy of Pediatrics. Healthy Children, Fit Children: Answers to Common Questions From Parents About Nutrition and Fitness. 2011.

[13] In the form of provitamin A carotenoids

[14] Products that bear the U.S. Food and Drug Administration (FDA) health claim for whole grains have at least 51 percent of the total ingredients by weight as whole-grain ingredients; they also meet other criteria.

[15] Foods that meet the whole grain-rich criteria for the school meal programs contain 100 percent whole grain or a blend of whole-grain meal and/or flour and enriched meal and/or flour of which at least 50 percent is whole grain. The remaining 50 percent or less of grains, if any, must be enriched. http://www.fns.usda.gov/sites/default/files/WholeGrainResource.pdf. Accessed October 22, 2015.

[16] Adapted from the Food Safety and Inspection Service (FSIS) guidance on whole-grain claims. Available at: http://www.fsis.usda.gov/wps/portal/fsis/home. Accessed November 25, 2015.

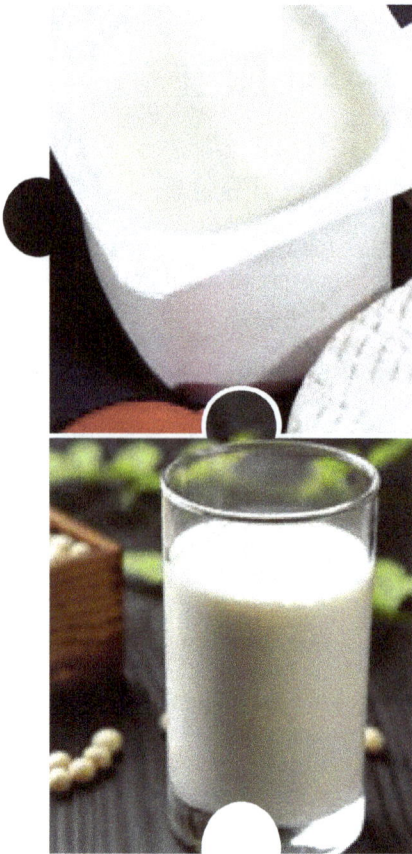

2 cup-equivalents per day for children ages 2 to 3 years, 2½ cup-equivalents per day for children ages 4 to 8 years, and 3 cup-equivalents per day for adolescents ages 9 to 18 years and for adults.

Key Nutrient Contributions: The dairy group contributes many nutrients, including calcium, phosphorus, vitamin A, vitamin D (in products fortified with vitamin D), riboflavin, vitamin B12, protein, potassium, zinc, choline, magnesium, and selenium.

Considerations: Fat-free and low-fat (1%) dairy products provide the same nutrients but less fat (and thus, fewer calories) than higher fat options, such as 2% and whole milk and regular cheese. Fat-free or low-fat milk and yogurt, in comparison to cheese, contain less saturated fats and sodium and more potassium, vitamin A, and vitamin D. Thus, increasing the proportion of dairy intake that is fat-free or low-fat milk or yogurt and decreasing the proportion that is cheese would decrease saturated fats and sodium and increase potassium, vitamin A, and vitamin D provided from the dairy group. Individuals who are lactose intolerant can choose low-lactose and lactose-free dairy products. Those who are unable or choose not to consume dairy products should consume foods that provide the range of nutrients generally obtained from dairy, including protein, calcium, potassium, magnesium, vitamin D, and vitamin A (e.g., fortified soy beverages [soymilk]). Additional sources of potassium, calcium, and vitamin D are found in Appendix 10, Appendix 11, and Appendix 12, respectively.

Dairy

Healthy Intake: Healthy eating patterns include fat-free and low-fat (1%) dairy, including milk, yogurt, cheese, or fortified soy beverages (commonly known as "soymilk"). Soy beverages fortified with calcium, vitamin A, and vitamin D, are included as part of the dairy group because they are similar to milk based on nutrient composition and in their use in meals. Other products sold as "milks" but made from plants (e.g., almond, rice, coconut, and hemp "milks") may contain calcium and be consumed as a source of calcium, but they are not included as part of the dairy group because their overall nutritional content is not similar to dairy milk and fortified soy beverages (soymilk). The recommended amounts of dairy in the Healthy U.S.-Style Pattern are based on age rather than calorie level and are

Protein Foods

Healthy Intake: Healthy eating patterns include a variety of protein foods in nutrient-dense forms. The protein foods group comprises a broad group of foods from both animal and plant sources and includes several subgroups: seafood; meats, poultry, and eggs; and nuts, seeds, and soy products. Legumes (beans and peas) may also be considered part of the protein foods group as well as the vegetables group (see the About Legumes (Beans and Peas) call-out box). Protein also is found in some foods from other food groups (e.g., dairy). The recommendation for protein foods in the Healthy U.S.-Style Eating Pattern at the 2,000-calorie level is 5½ ounce-equivalents of protein foods per day.

Key Nutrient Contributions: Protein foods are important sources of nutrients in addition to protein, including B vitamins (e.g., niacin, vitamin B_{12}, vitamin B_6, and riboflavin), selenium, choline, phosphorus, zinc, copper, vitamin D, and vitamin E). Nutrients provided by various types of protein foods differ. For example, meats provide the most zinc, while poultry provides the most niacin. Meats, poultry, and seafood provide heme iron, which is more bioavailable than the non-heme iron found in plant sources. Heme iron is especially important for young children and women who are capable of becoming pregnant or who are pregnant. Seafood provides the most vitamin B_{12} and vitamin D, in addition to almost all of the polyunsaturated omega-3 fatty acids, eicosapentaenoic acid (EPA), and docosahexaenoic acid (DHA), in the Patterns (see the About Seafood call-out box). Eggs provide the most choline, and nuts and seeds provide the most vitamin E. Soy products are a source of copper, manganese, and iron, as are legumes.

Considerations: For balance and flexibility within the food group, the Healthy U.S.-Style Eating Pattern includes weekly recommendations for the subgroups: seafood; meats, poultry, and eggs; and nuts, seeds, and soy products. A specific recommendation for at least 8 ounce-equivalents of seafood per week also is included for the 2,000-calorie level (see the About Seafood call-out box). One-half ounce of nuts or seeds counts as 1 ounce-equivalent of protein foods, and because they are high in calories, they should be eaten in small portions and used to replace other protein foods rather than being added to the diet. When selecting protein foods, nuts and seeds should be unsalted, and meats and poultry should be consumed in lean forms. Processed meats and processed poultry are sources of sodium and saturated fats, and intake of these products can be accommodated as long as sodium, saturated fats, added sugars, and total calories are within limits in the resulting eating pattern (see the About Meats and Poultry call-out box). The inclusion of protein foods from plants allows vegetarian options to be accommodated.

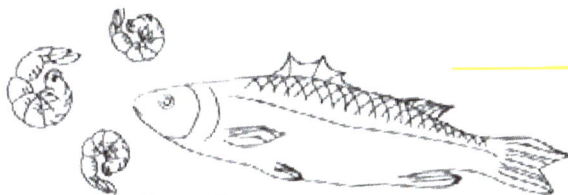

About Seafood

Seafood, which includes fish and shellfish, received particular attention in the *2010 Dietary Guidelines* because of evidence of health benefits for the general populations as well as for women who are pregnant or breastfeeding. For the general population, consumption of about 8 ounces per week of a variety of seafood, which provide an average consumption of 250 mg per day of EPA and DHA, is associated with reduced cardiac deaths among individuals with and without preexisting CVD. Similarly, consumption by women who are pregnant or breastfeeding of at least 8 ounces per week from seafood choices that are sources of DHA is associated with improved infant health outcomes.

The recommendation to consume 8 or more ounces per week (less for young children) of seafood is for the total package of nutrients that seafood provides, including its EPA and DHA content. Some seafood choices with higher amounts of EPA and DHA should be included.

Strong evidence from mostly prospective cohort studies but also randomized controlled trials has shown that eating patterns that include seafood are associated with reduced risk of CVD, and moderate evidence indicates that these eating patterns are associated with reduced risk of obesity. As described earlier, eating patterns consist of multiple, interacting food components and the relationships to health exist for the overall eating pattern, not necessarily to an isolated aspect of the diet.

Mercury is a heavy metal found in the form of methyl mercury in seafood in varying levels. Seafood choices higher in EPA and DHA but lower in methyl mercury are encouraged.[17] Seafood varieties commonly consumed in the United States that are higher in EPA and DHA and lower in methyl mercury include salmon, anchovies, herring, shad, sardines, Pacific oysters, trout, and Atlantic and Pacific mackerel (*not* king mackerel, which is high in methyl mercury). Individuals who regularly consume more than the recommended amounts of seafood that are in the Healthy U.S-Style Pattern should choose a mix of seafood that emphasizes choices relatively low in methyl mercury.

Some canned seafood, such as anchovies, may be high in sodium. To keep sodium intake below recommended limits, individuals can use the Nutrition Facts label to compare sodium amounts.

Women who are pregnant or breastfeeding should consume at least 8 and up to 12 ounces[18] of a variety of seafood per week, from choices that are lower in methyl mercury. Obstetricians and pediatricians should provide guidance on how to make healthy food choices that include seafood. Women who are pregnant or breastfeeding and young children should not eat certain types of fish that are high in methyl mercury.[19]

[17] State and local advisories provide information to guide consumers who eat fish caught from local waters. See the EPA website, "Fish Consumption Advisories, General Information." Available at: http://water.epa.gov/scitech/swguidance/fishshellfish/fishadvisories/general.cfm. Accessed September 26, 2015.

[18] Cooked, edible portion

[19] The U.S. Food and Drug Administration (FDA) and the U.S. Environmental Protection Agency (EPA) provide joint guidance regarding seafood consumption for women who are pregnant or breastfeeding and young children. For more information, see the FDA and EPA websites www.FDA.gov/fishadvice; www.EPA.gov/fishadvice.

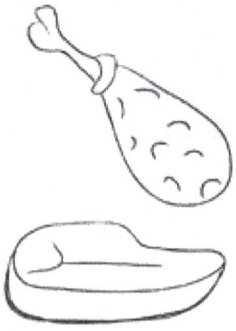

About Meats & Poultry

Meat, also known as red meat, includes all forms of beef, pork, lamb, veal, goat, and non-bird game (e.g., venison, bison, and elk). Poultry includes all forms of chicken, turkey, duck, geese, guineas, and game birds (e.g., quail and pheasant). Meats and poultry vary in fat content and include both fresh and processed forms. Lean meats and poultry contain less than 10 g of fat, 4.5 g or less of saturated fats, and less than 95 mg of cholesterol per 100 g and per labeled serving size (e.g., 95% lean ground beef, pork tenderloin, and skinless chicken or turkey breast). Processed meats and processed poultry (e.g., sausages, luncheon meats, bacon, and beef jerky) are products preserved by smoking, curing, salting, and/or the addition of chemical preservatives.

Strong evidence from mostly prospective cohort studies but also randomized controlled trials has shown that *eating patterns* that include lower intake of meats as well as processed meats and processed poultry are associated with reduced risk of CVD in adults. Moderate evidence indicates that these *eating patterns* are associated with reduced risk of obesity, type 2 diabetes, and some types of cancer in adults. As described earlier, eating patterns consist of multiple, interacting food components, and the relationships to health exist for the overall eating pattern, not necessarily to an isolated aspect of the diet. Much of this research on eating patterns has grouped together all meats and poultry, regardless of fat content or processing, though some evidence has identified lean meats and lean poultry in healthy eating patterns. In separate analyses, food pattern modeling has demonstrated that lean meats and lean poultry can contribute important nutrients within limits for sodium, calories from saturated fats and added sugars, and total calories when consumed in recommended amounts in healthy eating patterns, such as the Healthy U.S.-Style and Mediterranean-Style Eating Patterns.

The recommendation for the meats, poultry, and eggs subgroup in the Healthy U.S.-Style Eating Pattern at the 2,000-calorie level is 26 ounce-equivalents per week. This is the same as the amount that was in the primary USDA Food Patterns of the *2010 Dietary Guidelines*. As discussed in Chapter 2, average intakes of meats, poultry, and eggs for teen boys and adult men are above recommendations in the Healthy U.S.-Style Eating Pattern. For those who eat animal products, the recommendation for the protein foods subgroup of meats, poultry, and eggs can be met by consuming a variety of lean meats, lean poultry, and eggs. Choices within these eating patterns may include processed meats and processed poultry as long as the resulting eating pattern is within limits for sodium, calories from saturated fats and added sugars, and total calories.

Oils

Healthy Intake: Oils are fats that contain a high percentage of monounsaturated and polyunsaturated fats and are liquid at room temperature. Although they are not a food group, oils are emphasized as part of healthy eating patterns because they are the major source of essential fatty acids and vitamin E. Commonly consumed oils extracted from plants include canola, corn, olive, peanut, safflower, soybean, and sunflower oils. Oils also are naturally present in nuts, seeds, seafood, olives, and avocados. The fat in some tropical plants, such as coconut oil, palm kernel oil, and palm oil, are not included in the oils category because they do not resemble other oils in their composition. Specifically, they contain a higher percentage of saturated fats than other oils (see Dietary Fats: The Basics call-out box). The recommendation for oils in the Healthy U.S.-Style Eating Pattern at the 2,000-calorie level is 27 g (about 5 teaspoons) per day.

Key Nutrient Contributions: Oils provide essential fatty acids and vitamin E.

Considerations: Oils are part of healthy eating patterns, but because they are a concentrated source of calories, the amount consumed should be within the AMDR for total fats without exceeding calorie limits. Oils should replace solid fats rather than being added to the diet. More information on types of fats is provided in the Dietary Fats: The Basics call-out box, and information on the relationship between dietary fats and health is discussed in the Saturated Fats, *Trans* Fats, and Cholesterol section.

Dietary Fats: The Basics

Dietary fats are found in both plant and animal foods. They supply calories and help with the absorption of the fat-soluble vitamins A, D, E, and K. Some also are good sources of two essential fatty acids—linoleic acid and α-linolenic acid.

All dietary fats are composed of a mix of polyunsaturated, monounsaturated, and saturated fatty acids, in varied proportions (**Figure 1-2**). For example, most of the fatty acids in butter are saturated, but it also contains some monounsaturated and polyunsaturated fatty acids. Oils are mostly unsaturated fatty acids, though they have small amounts of saturated fatty acids.

Figure 1-2.
Fatty Acid Profiles of Common Fats & Oils

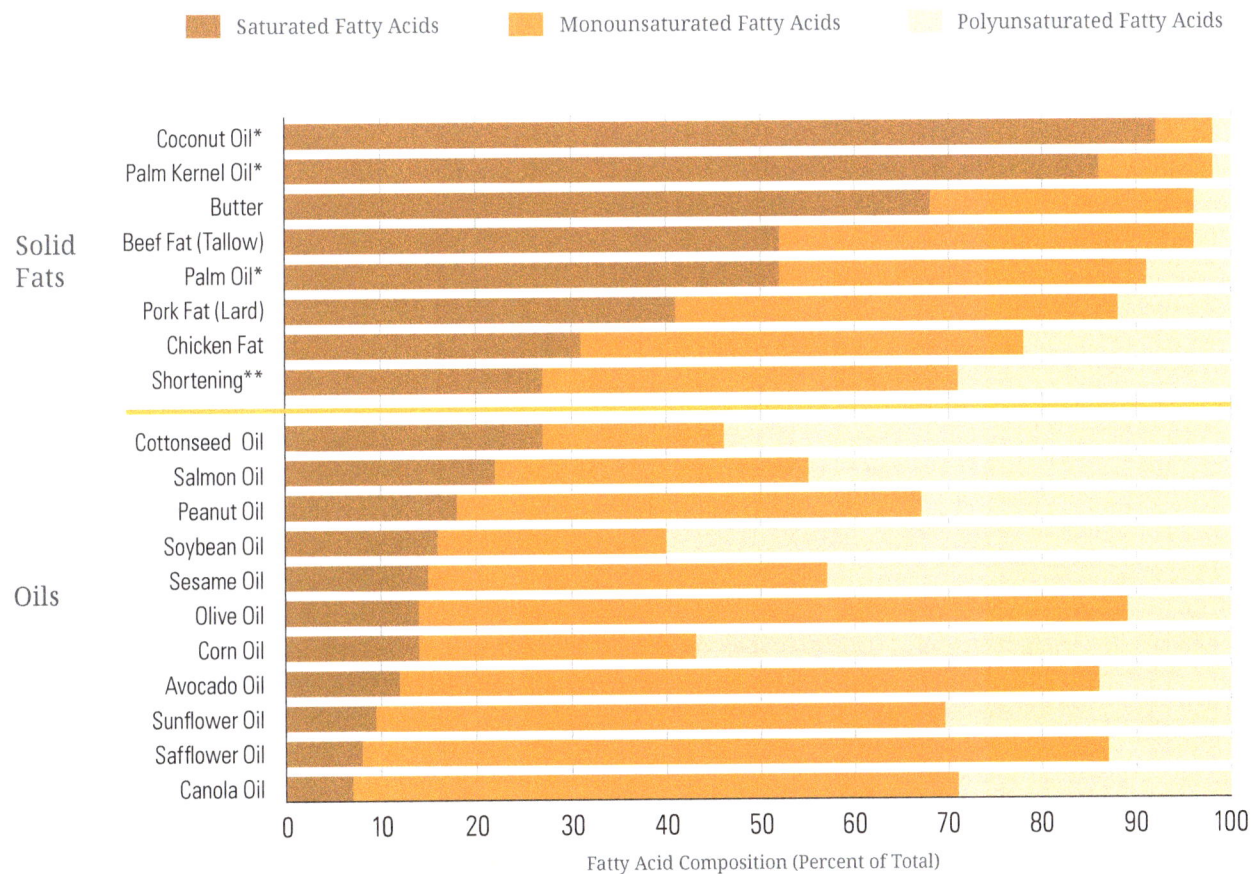

* Coconut, palm kernel, and palm oil are called oils because they come from plants. However, they are solid or semi-solid at room temperature due to their high content of short-chain saturated fatty acids. They are considered solid fats for nutritional purposes.

** Shortening may be made from partially hydrogenated vegetable oil, which contains *trans* fatty acids.

DATA SOURCES: U.S. Department of Agriculture, Agricultural Research Service, Nutrient Data Laboratory. USDA National Nutrient Database for Standard Reference. Release 27, 2015. Available at: http://ndb.nal.usda.gov/. Accessed August 31, 2015.

Dietary Fats: The Basics *(continued...)*

- **Polyunsaturated fatty acids (polyunsaturated fats[20])** are found in greatest amounts in sunflower, corn, soybean, and cottonseed oils; walnuts; pine nuts; and sesame, sunflower, pumpkin, and flax seeds. Only small amounts of polyunsaturated fats are found in most animal fats. Omega-3 (*n*-3) fatty acids are a type of polyunsaturated fats found in seafood, such as salmon, trout, herring, tuna, and mackerel, and in flax seeds and walnuts. EPA and DHA are long chain *n*-3 fatty acids found in seafood.

- **Monounsaturated fatty acids (monounsaturated fats)** are found in greatest amounts in olive, canola, peanut, sunflower, and safflower oils, and in avocados, peanut butter, and most nuts. Monounsaturated fats also are part of most animal fats such as fats from chicken, pork, beef, and wild game.

- **Saturated fatty acids (saturated fats)** are found in the greatest amounts in coconut and palm kernel oils, in butter and beef fats, and in palm oil. They also are found in other animal fats, such as pork and chicken fats and in other plant fats, such as nuts.

- ***Trans* fatty acids (*trans* fats)** are unsaturated fats found primarily in partially hydrogenated vegetable oils and foods containing these oils and in ruminant (animal) fats. They are structurally different from the unsaturated fatty acids that occur naturally in plant foods and differ in their health effects.

The proportions of fatty acids in a particular fat determine the physical form of the fat:

- Fats with a higher amount of polyunsaturated and monounsaturated fatty acids are usually liquid at room temperature and are referred to as "oils."

- Fats with a higher amount of saturated fatty acids are usually solid at room temperature and are referred to as "solid fats." Fats containing *trans* fatty acids are also classified as solid fats, although they may or may not be solid at room temperature.

A relevant detail in the complexity of making food-based recommendations that consider nutrients is the difference between the terms "saturated fats" and "solid fats." Although they are closely related terms, saturated fats and solid fats are not synonymous. The term "saturated fats" refers to saturated fatty acids, a nutrient found in foods, while the term "solid fats" describes the physical manifestation of the fats in a food. Some solid fats, such as the strip of fat around a piece of meat, can easily be seen. Other solid fats are not so visible. For example, the solid fats in whole milk are suspended in the fluid milk by the process of homogenization.

Margarines and margarine-like vegetable oil spreads are food products composed of one or more oils or solid fats designed to replace butter, which is high in saturated fats. These products may be sold in sticks, tubs, bottles, or sprays. Margarine and vegetable oil spreads generally contain less saturated fats than butter. However, they vary in their total fat and calorie content and in the fat and oil blends used to make them and, thus, in the proportions of saturated, unsaturated, and *trans* fats they contain. It is important to read the Nutrition Facts label to identify the calorie and saturated and *trans* fats content of the spread and choose foods with no *trans* fats and lower amounts of saturated fats.

The *Dietary Guidelines* provides recommendations on saturated fats as well as on solid fats because its aim is to improve the health of the U.S. population through food-based guidance. It includes recommendations on saturated fats because of the strong relationship of this nutrient to a health outcome (CVD risk). It includes recommendations on solid fats because, as discussed in Chapter 2, they are abundant in the diets of the U.S. population, and reducing solid fats when making food choices is an important way to reduce saturated fats and excess calories.

[20] The term "fats" rather than "fatty acids" is generally used in this document when discussing categories of fatty acids (e.g., unsaturated, saturated, trans) for consistency with the Nutrition Facts label and other Federal materials.

Limits on Calories That Remain After Food Group Needs Are Met in Nutrient-Dense Forms

The USDA Food Patterns are designed to meet food group and nutrient recommendations while staying within calorie needs. To achieve this goal, the Patterns are based on consuming foods in their nutrient-dense forms (i.e., without added sugars and in the leanest and lowest fat forms, see Appendix 6). For nearly all calorie levels, most of the calories in the USDA Food Patterns are needed for nutrient-dense food choices, and only a limited number remain for other uses. These calories are indicated in the USDA Food Patterns as "limits on calories for other uses." For example, after food group needs are met in the Healthy U.S.-Style Eating Pattern from 1,000 to 1,600 calories, only 100 to 170 calories per day remain within the limit for other uses. In the 2,000-calorie pattern, the limit for other uses is 270 calories and in the 2,800-calorie pattern, 400 calories (see Appendix 3, Appendix 4, and Appendix 5). Calories up to the limit for the specific pattern can be used to eat foods that are not in nutrient-dense forms (e.g., to accommodate calories from added sugars, added refined starches, or solid fats) or to eat more than the recommended amount of nutrient-dense foods. If alcohol is consumed, calories from alcoholic beverages should also be accounted for within this limit to keep total calorie intake at an appropriate level.

As discussed in Chapter 2, in contrast to the healthy choices that make up the Patterns, foods from most food groups as they are typically consumed in the United States are not in nutrient-dense forms. In addition, foods and beverages are consumed that are primarily composed of added sugars and/or solid fats, and provide excess calories without contributing to meeting food group recommendations. The excess calories consumed from these sources far exceed the limited number of calories available for choices other than nutrient-dense foods in each food group.

From a public health perspective, it is important to identify the calories that are needed to meet food group needs to help inform guidance on limits from calories from added sugars, solid fats, alcohol[21], or other sources, in order to help individuals move toward healthy eating patterns within calorie limits. The USDA Food Patterns can be used to plan and serve meals for individuals, households, and in a variety of organizational settings (e.g., schools, worksites, and other community settings). The limit on calories for other uses can assist in determining how to plan and select foods that can fit within healthy eating patterns, such as how many calories are available to select foods from a food group that are not in nutrient-dense forms. As discussed in the next portion of the chapter, additional constraints apply related to other dietary components when building healthy eating patterns.

Other Dietary Components

In addition to the food groups, it is important to consider other food components when making food and beverage choices. The components discussed here include added sugars, saturated fats, *trans* fats, cholesterol, sodium, alcohol, and caffeine. For each component, information is provided on how the component relates to eating patterns and outlines considerations related to the component. See Chapter 2 for a further discussion of each of these components, current intakes, and shifts that are needed to help individuals align with a healthy eating pattern.

Added Sugars

Healthy Intake: Added sugars include syrups and other caloric sweeteners. When sugars are added to foods and beverages to sweeten them, they add calories without contributing essential nutrients. Consumption of added sugars can make it difficult for individuals to meet their nutrient needs while staying within calorie limits. Naturally occurring sugars, such as those in fruit or milk, are not added sugars. Specific examples of added sugars that can be listed as an ingredient include brown sugar, corn sweetener, corn syrup, dextrose, fructose, glucose, high-fructose corn syrup, honey, invert sugar, lactose, malt syrup, maltose, molasses, raw sugar, sucrose, trehalose, and turbinado sugar.

Healthy eating patterns limit added sugars to less than 10 percent of calories per day. This recommendation is a target to help the public achieve a healthy eating pattern, which means meeting nutrient and food group needs through nutrient-dense food and beverage choices and staying within calorie limits. When added sugars in foods and beverages exceed 10 percent of calories, a healthy eating pattern may be difficult to achieve. This target also is informed by national data on intakes of calories from added sugars, which as discussed in Chapter 2, account on average for almost 270 calories, or more than 13 percent of calories per day in the U.S. population.

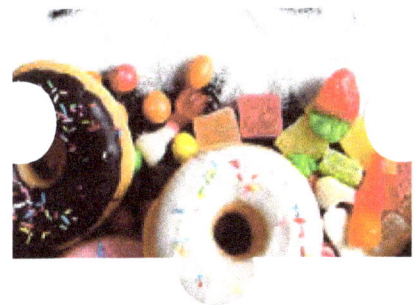

[21] It is not recommended that individuals begin drinking or drink more for any reason. The amount of alcohol and calories in beverages varies and should be accounted for within the limits of healthy eating patterns. Alcohol should be consumed only by adults of legal drinking age. There are many circumstances in which individuals should not drink, such as during pregnancy. See Appendix 9. Alcohol for additional information.

2015-2020 Dietary Guidelines for Americans • Chapter 1 — Page 28

Figure 1-3.

Hidden Components in Eating Patterns

Many of the foods and beverages we eat contain sodium, saturated fats, and added sugars. Making careful choices, as in this example, keeps amounts of these components within their limits while meeting nutrient needs to achieve a healthy eating pattern.

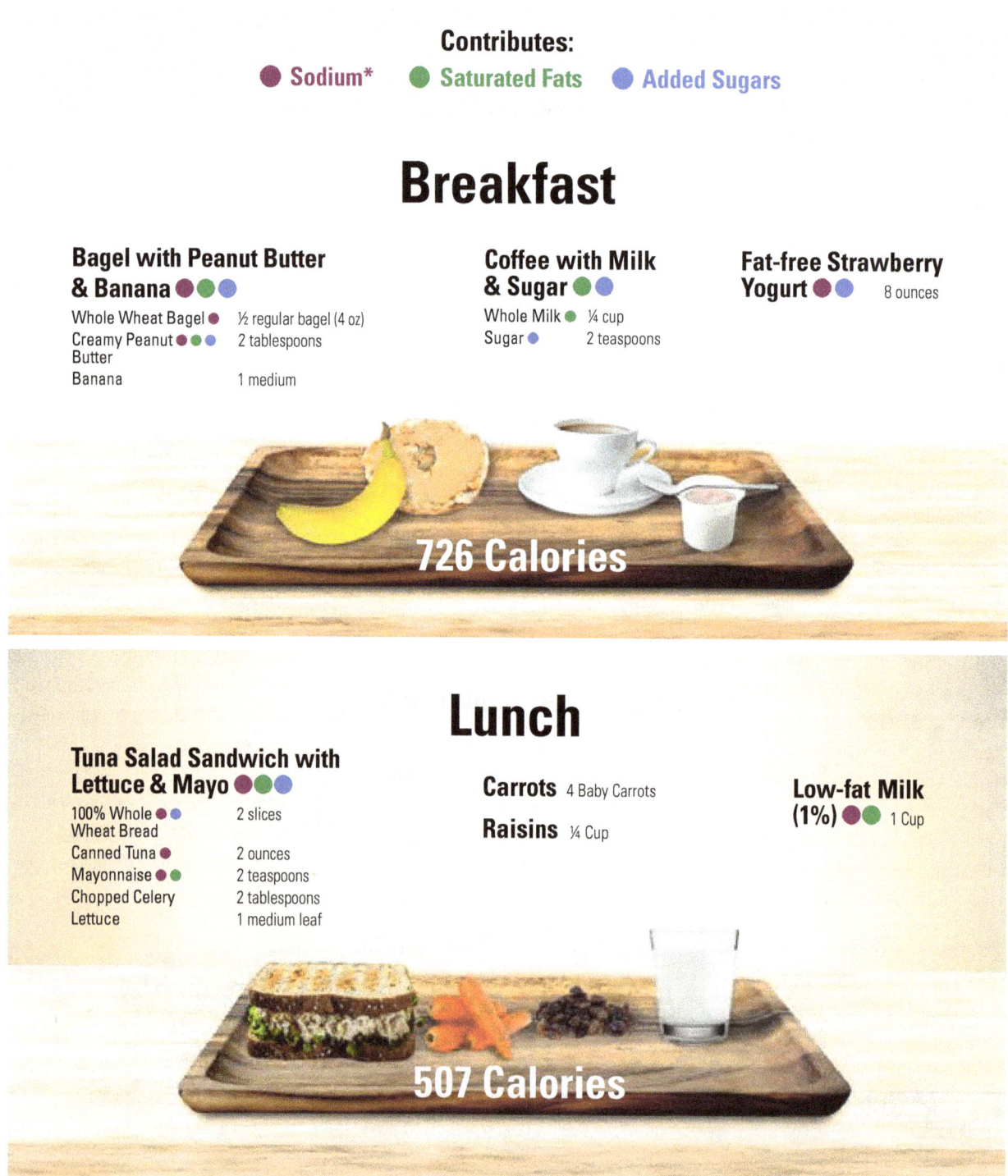

Contributes:

● Sodium*   ● Saturated Fats   ● Added Sugars

Breakfast

Bagel with Peanut Butter & Banana ●●●

Whole Wheat Bagel ●	½ regular bagel (4 oz)
Creamy Peanut Butter ●●●	2 tablespoons
Banana	1 medium

Coffee with Milk & Sugar ●●

Whole Milk ●	¼ cup
Sugar ●	2 teaspoons

Fat-free Strawberry Yogurt ●●   8 ounces

726 Calories

Lunch

Tuna Salad Sandwich with Lettuce & Mayo ●●●

100% Whole Wheat Bread ●●	2 slices
Canned Tuna ●	2 ounces
Mayonnaise ●●	2 teaspoons
Chopped Celery	2 tablespoons
Lettuce	1 medium leaf

Carrots 4 Baby Carrots

Raisins ¼ Cup

Low-fat Milk (1%) ●● 1 Cup

507 Calories

Foods very low in sodium not marked

Contributes:

● **Sodium***   ● **Saturated Fats**   ● Added Sugars

Dinner

Spaghetti & Meatballs ●●●

Spaghetti	1 cup, cooked
Spaghetti Sauce ●●	¼ cup
Diced Tomatoes (canned, no salt added)	¼ cup
Meatballs ●●	3 medium meatballs
Parmesan Cheese ●●	1 tablespoon

Apple, Raw ½ medium

Water, Tap 1 cup

Garden Salad ●●●

Mixed Greens	1 cup
Cucumber	3 slices
Avocado ●	¼ cup, cubed
Garbanzo Beans ● (canned, low sodium)	¼ cup
Cheddar Cheese ● (reduced fat)	3 tablespoons, shredded
Ranch Salad Dressing ●●●	1 tablespoon

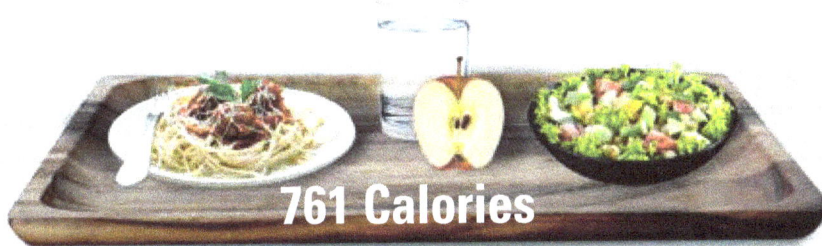

761 Calories

Total

Sodium: 2,253 mg
less than or equal to 2,300 mg

Calories From Saturated Fats: 153 (8% of Total Calories)
less than or equal to 10% of calories

Calories From Added Sugars: 164 (8% of Total Calories)
less than or equal to 10% of calories

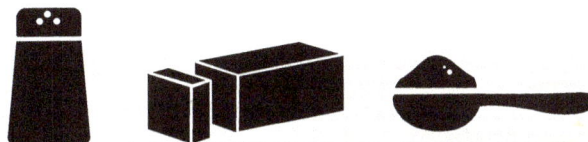

1,995 Calories

* Foods very low in sodium not marked

The USDA Food Patterns show that an eating pattern with enough foods from all food groups to meet nutrient needs without eating too many calories has only limited room for calories from added sugars. At most lower calorie levels (i.e., 1,200 to 1,800 calories), the calories that remain after meeting food group recommendations in nutrient-dense forms ("limits on calories for other uses") are less than 10 percent per day of calories; however, at higher calorie levels, the limits on calories for other uses are more than 10 percent per day. The recommendation to limit added sugars to no more than 10 percent of calories is a target that applies to all calorie levels to help individuals move toward healthy eating patterns within calorie limits.

Although the evidence for added sugars and health outcomes is still developing, the recommendation to limit calories from added sugars is consistent with research examining *eating patterns* and health. Strong evidence from mostly prospective cohort studies but also randomized controlled trials has shown that *eating patterns* that include lower intake of sources of added sugars are associated with reduced risk of CVD in adults, and moderate evidence indicates that these *eating patterns* are associated with reduced risk of obesity, type 2 diabetes, and some types of cancer in adults. As described earlier, eating patterns consist of multiple, interacting food components, and the relationships to health exist for the overall eating pattern, not necessarily to an isolated aspect of the diet. Moderate evidence indicates a relationship between added sugars and dental caries in children and adults.

Considerations: Added sugars provide sweetness that can help improve the palatability of foods, help with preservation, and/or contribute to functional attributes such as viscosity, texture, body, color,

and browning capability. As discussed in Chapter 2, the two main sources of added sugars in U.S. diets are sugar-sweetened beverages and snacks and sweets. Many foods high in calories from added sugars provide few or no essential nutrients or dietary fiber and, therefore, may contribute to excess calorie intake without contributing to diet quality; intake of these foods should be limited to help achieve healthy eating patterns within calorie limits. There is room for Americans to include limited amounts of added sugars in their eating patterns, including to improve the palatability of some nutrient-dense foods, such as fruits and vegetables that are naturally tart (e.g., cranberries and rhubarb). Healthy eating patterns can accommodate other nutrient-dense foods with small amounts of added sugars, such as whole-grain breakfast cereals or fat-free yogurt, as long as calories from added sugars do not exceed 10 percent per day, total carbohydrate intake remains within the AMDR, and total calorie intake remains within limits.

It should be noted that replacing added sugars with high-intensity sweeteners may reduce calorie intake in the short-term, yet questions remain about their effectiveness as a long-term weight management strategy. High-intensity sweeteners that have been approved by the U.S. Food and Drug Administration (FDA) include saccharin, aspartame, acesulfame potassium (Ace-K), and sucralose.[22] Based on the available scientific evidence, these high-intensity sweeteners have been determined to be safe for the general population. This means that there is reasonable certainty of no harm under the intended conditions of use because the estimated daily intake is not expected to exceed the acceptable daily intake for each sweetener. The FDA has determined that the estimated daily intake of these high-intensity sweeteners would

not exceed the acceptable daily intake, even for high consumers of each substance.

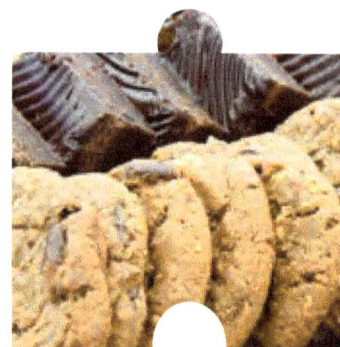

Saturated Fats, *Trans* Fats, & Cholesterol

Saturated Fats

Healthy Intake: Intake of saturated fats should be limited to less than 10 percent of calories per day by replacing them with unsaturated fats and while keeping total dietary fats within the age-appropriate AMDR. The human body uses some saturated fats for physiological and structural functions, but it makes more than enough to meet those needs. Individuals 2 years and older therefore have no dietary requirement for saturated fats.

Strong and consistent evidence shows that replacing saturated fats with unsaturated fats, especially polyunsaturated fats, is associated with reduced blood levels of total cholesterol and of low-density lipoprotein-cholesterol (LDL-cholesterol). Additionally, strong and consistent evidence shows that replacing saturated fats with polyunsaturated fats is associated with a reduced risk of CVD events (heart attacks) and CVD-related deaths.

Some evidence has shown that replacing saturated fats with plant sources of monounsaturated fats, such as olive oil and nuts, may be associated with a reduced risk of CVD. However, the evidence base

[22] For more information, see: FDA. High-Intensity Sweeteners. May 19, 2014. [Updated November 5, 2014.] Available at: http://www.fda.gov/food/ingredientspackaginglabeling/foodadditivesingredients/ucm397716.htm. Accessed October 19, 2015. This page provides a link to "Additional Information about High-Intensity Sweeteners Permitted for use in Food in the United States" which includes more information on types and uses of high-intensity sweeteners and the scientific evidence evaluated by the FDA for safety for the general population.

for monounsaturated fats is not as strong as the evidence base for replacement with polyunsaturated fats. Evidence has also shown that replacing saturated fats with carbohydrates reduces blood levels of total and LDL-cholesterol, but increases blood levels of triglycerides and reduces high-density lipoprotein-cholesterol (HDL-cholesterol). Replacing total fat or saturated fats with carbohydrates is not associated with reduced risk of CVD. Additional research is needed to determine whether this relationship is consistent across categories of carbohydrates (e.g., whole versus refined grains; intrinsic versus added sugars), as they may have different associations with various health outcomes. Therefore, saturated fats in the diet should be replaced with polyunsaturated and monounsaturated fats.

Considerations: As discussed in Chapter 2, the main sources of saturated fats in the U.S. diet include mixed dishes containing cheese, meat, or both, such as burgers, sandwiches, and tacos; pizza; rice, pasta, and grain dishes; and meat, poultry, and seafood dishes. Although some saturated fats are inherent in foods, others are added. Healthy eating patterns can accommodate nutrient-dense foods with small amounts of saturated fats, as long as calories from saturated fats do not exceed 10 percent per day, intake of total fats remains within the AMDR, and total calorie intake remains within limits. When possible, foods high in saturated fats should be replaced with foods high in unsaturated fats, and other choices to reduce solid fats should be made (see Chapter 2).

Trans Fats

Individuals should limit intake of *trans* fats to as low as possible by limiting foods that contain synthetic sources of *trans* fats, such as partially hydrogenated oils in margarines, and by limiting other solid fats. A number of studies have observed an association between increased intake of *trans* fats and increased risk of CVD. This increased risk is due, in part, to its LDL-cholesterol-raising effect.

Trans fats occur naturally in some foods and also are produced in a process called hydrogenation. Hydrogenation is used by food manufacturers to make products containing unsaturated fatty acids solid at room temperature (i.e., more saturated) and therefore more resistant to becoming spoiled or rancid. Partial hydrogenation means that some, but not all, unsaturated fatty acids are converted to saturated fatty acids; some of the unsaturated fatty acids are changed from a *cis* to *trans* configuration. *Trans* fatty acids produced this way are referred to as "artificial" or "industrially produced" trans fatty acids. Artificial *trans* fatty acids are found in the partially hydrogenated oils[23] used in some margarines, snack foods, and prepared desserts as a replacement for saturated fatty acids. Although food manufacturers and restaurants have reduced the amounts of artificial *trans* fats in many foods in recent years, these fats can still be found in some processed foods, such as some desserts, microwave popcorn, frozen pizza, margarines, and coffee creamers.

Naturally occurring *trans* fats, known as "natural" or "ruminant" *trans* fats, are produced by ruminant animals. Natural *trans* fats are present in small quantities in dairy products and meats, and consuming fat-free or low-fat dairy products and lean meats and poultry will reduce the intake of natural *trans* fats from these foods. Because natural *trans* fats are present in dairy products and meats in only small quantities and these foods can be important sources of nutrients, these foods do not need to be eliminated from the diet.

Dietary Cholesterol

The body uses cholesterol for physiological and structural functions but makes more than enough for these purposes. Therefore, people do not need to obtain cholesterol through foods.

The Key Recommendation from the *2010 Dietary Guidelines* to limit consumption of dietary cholesterol to 300 mg per day is not included in the 2015 edition, but this change does not suggest that dietary cholesterol is no longer important to consider when building healthy eating patterns. As recommended by the IOM,[24] individuals should eat as little dietary cholesterol as possible while consuming a healthy eating pattern. In general, foods that are higher in dietary cholesterol, such as fatty meats and high-fat dairy products, are also higher in saturated fats. The USDA Food Patterns are limited in saturated fats, and because of the commonality of food sources of saturated fats and dietary cholesterol, the Patterns are also low in dietary cholesterol. For example, the Healthy U.S.-Style Eating Pattern contains approximately 100 to 300 mg of cholesterol across the 12 calorie levels. Current average intake of dietary cholesterol among those 1 year and older in the United States is approximately 270 mg per day.

Strong evidence from mostly prospective cohort studies but also randomized controlled trials has shown that *eating patterns* that include lower intake of dietary cholesterol are associated with reduced risk of CVD, and moderate evidence indicates that these eating patterns are associated with reduced risk of obesity. As described earlier, *eating patterns* consist of multiple, interacting food components and the relationships to health exist for the overall *eating pattern*, not necessarily to an isolated aspect of the diet. More research is needed

---

[23] The FDA has determined that partially hydrogenated oils, which are the primary dietary source of industrially produced trans fats, are no longer generally recognized as safe (GRAS), with compliance expected by June 18, 2018. FDA. Final Determination Regarding Partially Hydrogenated Oils. Federal Register. June 17, 2015;80(116):34650-34670. Available at: https://www.federalregister.gov/articles/2015/06/17/2015-14883/final-determination-regarding-partially-hydrogenated-oils. Accessed October 20, 2015.

[24] Institute of Medicine. Dietary Reference Intakes for Energy, Carbohydrate, Fiber, Fat, Fatty Acids, Cholesterol, Protein, and Amino Acids. Washington (DC): The National Academies Press; 2002.

Dietary Approaches to Stop Hypertension (DASH)

The DASH dietary pattern is an example of a healthy eating pattern and has many of the same characteristics as the Healthy U.S.-Style Eating Pattern. The DASH dietary pattern and several variations have been tested in randomized controlled clinical trials to study the effect of the DASH dietary pattern on CVD risk factors. The original DASH trial demonstrated that the DASH dietary pattern lowered blood pressure and LDL-cholesterol levels, resulting in reduced CVD risk, compared to diets that resembled a typical American diet. The DASH-Sodium trial confirmed the beneficial blood pressure and LDL-cholesterol effects of the DASH eating pattern at three levels of dietary sodium intake and also demonstrated a step-wise lowering of blood pressure as sodium intake was reduced. The OmniHeart Trial found that replacing some of the carbohydrates in DASH with the same amount of either protein or unsaturated fats lowered blood pressure and LDL-cholesterol levels more than the original DASH dietary pattern.

The DASH Eating Plan is high in vegetables, fruits, low-fat dairy products, whole grains, poultry, fish, beans, and nuts and is low in sweets, sugar-sweetened beverages, and red meats. It is low in saturated fats and rich in potassium, calcium, and magnesium, as well as dietary fiber and protein. It also is lower in sodium than the typical American diet, and includes menus with two levels of sodium, 2,300 and 1,500 mg per day. Additional details on DASH are available at http://www.nhlbi.nih.gov/health/health-topics/topics/dash.

Caffeine

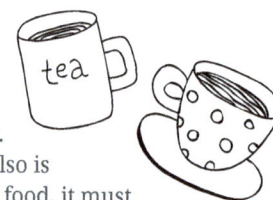

Caffeine is not a nutrient; it is a dietary component that functions in the body as a stimulant. Caffeine occurs naturally in plants (e.g., coffee beans, tea leaves, cocoa beans, kola nuts). It also is added to foods and beverages (e.g., caffeinated soda, energy drinks). If caffeine is added to a food, it must be included in the listing of ingredients on the food label.[25] Most intake of caffeine in the United States comes from coffee, tea, and soda. Caffeinated beverages vary widely in their caffeine content. Caffeinated coffee beverages include drip/brewed coffee (12 mg/fl oz), instant coffee (8 mg/fl oz), espresso (64 mg/fl oz), and specialty beverages made from coffee or espresso, such as cappuccinos and lattes. Amounts of caffeine in other beverages such as brewed black tea (6 mg/fl oz), brewed green tea (2-5 mg/fl oz), and caffeinated soda[26] (1-4 mg/fl oz) also vary. Beverages within the energy drinks category have the greatest variability (3-35 mg/fl oz).

Much of the available evidence on caffeine focuses on coffee intake. Moderate coffee consumption (three to five 8-oz cups/day or providing up to 400 mg/day of caffeine) can be incorporated into healthy eating patterns. This guidance on coffee is informed by strong and consistent evidence showing that, in healthy adults, moderate coffee consumption is not associated with an increased risk of major chronic diseases (e.g., cancer) or premature death, especially from CVD. However, individuals who do not consume caffeinated coffee or other caffeinated beverages are not encouraged to incorporate them into their eating pattern. Limited and mixed evidence is available from randomized controlled trials examining the relationship between those energy drinks which have high caffeine content and cardiovascular risk factors and other health outcomes. In addition, caffeinated beverages, such as some sodas or energy drinks, may include calories from added sugars, and although coffee itself has minimal calories, coffee beverages often contain added calories from cream, whole or 2% milk, creamer, and added sugars, which should be limited. The same considerations apply to calories added to tea or other similar beverages.

Those who choose to drink alcohol should be cautious about mixing caffeine and alcohol together or consuming them at the same time; see Appendix 9. Alcohol for additional discussion. In addition, women who are capable of becoming pregnant or who are trying to, or who are pregnant, and those who are breastfeeding should consult their health care providers for advice concerning caffeine consumption.

[25] Some dietary supplements such as energy shots also contain caffeine, but the amount of caffeine in these products is not required to be disclosed

[26] Caffeine is a substance that is generally recognized as safe (GRAS) in cola-type beverages by the U.S. Food and Drug Administration for use by adults and children. Code of Federal Regulation Title 21, Subchapter B, Part 182, Subpart B. Caffeine. U.S. Government Printing Office. November 23, 2015. Available at: http://www.ecfr.gov/cgi-bin/retrieveECFR?gp=1&SID=f8c3068e9ec0062a3b4078cfa6361cf6&ty=HTML&h=L&mc=true&r=SECTION&n=se21.3.182_11180.

regarding the dose-response relationship between dietary cholesterol and blood cholesterol levels. Adequate evidence is not available for a quantitative limit for dietary cholesterol specific to the *Dietary Guidelines*.

Dietary cholesterol is found only in animal foods such as egg yolk, dairy products, shellfish, meats, and poultry. A few foods, notably egg yolks and some shellfish, are higher in dietary cholesterol but not saturated fats. Eggs and shellfish can be consumed along with a variety of other choices within and across the subgroup recommendations of the protein foods group.

Sodium

Healthy Intake: The scientific consensus from expert bodies, such as the IOM, the American Heart Association, and Dietary Guidelines Advisory Committees, is that average sodium intake, which is currently 3,440 mg per day (see Chapter 2), is too high and should be reduced. Healthy eating patterns limit sodium to less than 2,300 mg per day for adults and children ages 14 years and older and to the age- and sex-appropriate Tolerable Upper Intake Levels (UL) of sodium for children younger than 14 years (see Appendix 7). Sodium is an essential nutrient and is needed by the body in relatively small quantities, provided that substantial sweating does not occur.[27] Sodium is primarily consumed as salt (sodium chloride).

The limits for sodium are the age- and sex-appropriate ULs. The UL is the highest daily nutrient intake level that is likely to pose no risk of adverse health effects to almost all individuals in the general population. The recommendation for adults and children ages 14 years and older to limit sodium intake to less than 2,300 mg per day is based on evidence showing a linear dose-response relationship between increased sodium intake and increased blood pressure in adults. In addition, moderate evidence suggests an association between increased sodium intake and increased risk of CVD in adults. However, this evidence is not as consistent as the evidence on blood pressure, a surrogate indicator of CVD risk.

Calorie intake is highly associated with sodium intake (i.e., the more foods and beverages people consume, the more sodium they tend to consume). Because children have lower calorie needs than adults, the IOM established lower ULs for children younger than 14 years of age based on median intake of calories. Similar to adults, moderate evidence also indicates that the linear dose-response relationship between sodium intake and blood pressure is found in children as well.

Adults with prehypertension and hypertension would particularly benefit from blood pressure lowering. For these individuals, further reduction to 1,500 mg per day can result in even greater blood pressure reduction. Because of the linear dose-response relationship between sodium intake and blood pressure, every incremental decrease in sodium intake that moves toward recommended limits is encouraged. Even without reaching the limits for sodium intake, strong evidence indicates that reductions in sodium intake can lower blood pressure among people with prehypertension and hypertension. Further, strong evidence has demonstrated that adults who would benefit from blood pressure lowering should combine the Dietary Approaches to Stop Hypertension (DASH) dietary pattern with lower sodium intake (see Dietary Approaches to Stop Hypertension call-out box).

Considerations: As a food ingredient, sodium has multiple uses, such as in curing meat, baking, thickening, enhancing flavor (including the flavor of other ingredients), as a preservative, and in retaining moisture. For example, some fresh meats have sodium solutions added to help retain moisture in cooking. As discussed in Chapter 2, sodium is found in foods across the food supply, including mixed dishes such as burgers, sandwiches, and tacos; rice, pasta, and grain dishes; pizza; meat, poultry, and seafood dishes; and soups. Multiple strategies should be implemented to reduce sodium intake to the recommended limits (see Chapter 3. Everyone Has a Role in Supporting Healthy Eating Patterns).

Alcohol

Alcohol is not a component of the USDA Food Patterns. The *Dietary Guidelines* does not recommend that individuals who do not drink alcohol start drinking for any reason. If alcohol is consumed, it should be in moderation—up to one drink per day for women and up to two drinks per day for men—and only by adults of legal drinking age.[6] There are also many circumstances in which individuals should not drink, such as during pregnancy. For the purposes of evaluating amounts of alcohol that may be consumed, the *Dietary Guidelines* includes drink-equivalents. One alcoholic drink-equivalent is described as containing 14 g (0.6 fl oz) of pure alcohol. [28] The following are reference beverages that are one alcoholic drink-equivalent: 12 fluid ounces of regular beer (5% alcohol), 5 fluid ounces of wine (12% alcohol), or 1.5 fluid ounces of 80 proof distilled spirits (40% alcohol).[29] The amount of alcohol and calories in beverages varies and should be accounted for within the limits of healthy eating patterns so that calorie limits are not exceeded. See Appendix 9. Alcohol for additional information.

---

[27] The IOM set an Adequate Intake (AI) level for sodium to meet the sodium needs of healthy and moderately active individuals. Because of increased loss of sodium from sweat, the AI does not apply to highly active individuals and workers exposed to extreme heat stress, estimated to be less than 1 percent of the U.S. population. Institute of Medicine. Dietary Reference Intakes for Water, Potassium, Sodium, Chloride, and Sulfate. Washington (DC): The National Academies Press; 2005.

[28] Bowman SA, Clemens JC, Friday JE, Thoerig RC, and Moshfegh AJ. 2014. Food Patterns Equivalents Database 2011-12: Methodology and User Guide [Online]. Food Surveys Research Group, Beltsville Human Nutrition Research Center, Agricultural Research Service, U.S. Department of Agriculture, Beltsville, Maryland. Available at: http://www.ars.usda.gov/nea/bhnrc/fsrg. Accessed November 3, 2015. For additional information, see the National Institute on Alcohol Abuse and Alcoholism (NIAAA) webpage available at: http://rethinkingdrinking.niaaa.nih.gov/.

[29] Drink-equivalents are not intended to serve as a standard drink definition for regulatory purposes.

Examples of Other Healthy Eating Patterns

The U.S. population consumes many different styles of eating patterns other than the "typical American pattern" that provides the basis for the Healthy U.S.-Style Eating Pattern (see Appendix 3 and Table 1-1). There are many ways to consume a healthy eating pattern, and the evidence to support multiple approaches has expanded over time. The Healthy Mediterranean-Style Eating Pattern and Healthy Vegetarian Eating Pattern, which were developed by modifying the Healthy U.S.-Style Eating Pattern, are two examples of healthy eating patterns individuals may choose based on personal preference. Similar to the Healthy U.S.-Style Eating Pattern, these patterns were designed to consider the types and proportions of foods Americans typically consume, but in nutrient-dense forms and appropriate amounts, which result in eating patterns that are attainable and relevant in the U.S. population. Additionally, healthy eating patterns can be flexible with respect to the intake of carbohydrate, protein, and fat within the context of the AMDR.[30]

As with the Healthy U.S.-Style Eating Pattern, each provides recommended intakes at 12 different calorie levels (see Appendix 4 and Appendix 5). The 2,000 calorie level for each Pattern is shown here as an example (Table 1-2).

Healthy Mediterranean-Style Eating Pattern

A Healthy Mediterranean-Style Eating Pattern (Appendix 4) was designed by modifying the Healthy U.S.-Style Eating

[30] Institute of Medicine. Dietary Reference Intakes for Energy, Carbohydrate, Fiber, Fat, Fatty Acids, Cholesterol, Protein, and Amino Acids. Washington (DC): The National Academies Press; 2002.

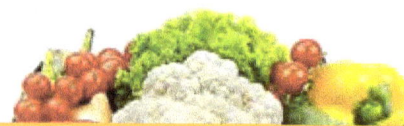

Table 1-2.

Composition of the Healthy Mediterranean-Style & Healthy Vegetarian Eating Patterns at the 2,000-Calorie Level,[a] With Daily or Weekly Amounts From Food Groups, Subgroups, & Components

Food Group[b]	Healthy Mediterranean-Style Eating Pattern	Healthy Vegetarian Eating Pattern
Vegetables	**2½ c-eq/day**	**2½ c-eq/day**
Dark Green	1½ c-eq/week	1½ c-eq/week
Red & Orange	5½ c-eq/week	5½ c-eq/week
Legumes (Beans & Peas)	1½ c-eq/week	3 c-eq/week[c]
Starchy	5 c-eq/week	5 c-eq/week
Other	4 c-eq/week	4 c-eq/week
Fruits	**2½ c-eq/day**	**2 c-eq/day**
Grains	**6 oz-eq/day**	**6½ oz-eq/day**
Whole Grains	≥3 oz-eq/day	≥3½ oz-eq/day
Refined Grains	≤3 oz-eq/day	≤3 oz-eq/day
Dairy	**2 c-eq/day**	**3 c-eq/day**
Protein Foods	**6½ oz-eq/day**	**3½ oz-eq/day[c]**
Seafood	15 oz-eq/week[d]	—
Meats, Poultry, Eggs	26 oz-eq/week	3 oz-eq/week (eggs)
Nuts, Seeds, Soy Products	5 oz-eq/week	14 oz-eq/week
Oils	**27 g/day**	**27 g/day**
Limit on Calories for Other Uses (% of Calories)[e]	**260 kcal/day (13%)**	**290 kcal/day (15%)**

[a] Food group amounts shown in cup- (c) or ounce- (oz) equivalents (eq). Oils are shown in grams (g). Quantity equivalents for each food group are defined in Appendix 3. Amounts will vary for those who need less than 2,000 or more than 2,000 calories per day. See Appendix 4 and Appendix 5 for all 12 calorie levels of the patterns.

[b] Definitions for each food group and subgroup are provided throughout the chapter and are compiled in Appendix 3.

[c] Vegetarian patterns include 1½ cups per week of legumes as a vegetable subgroup, and an additional 6 oz-eq (1½ cups) per week of legumes as a protein food. The total amount is shown here as legumes in the vegetable group.

[d] The FDA and EPA provide additional guidance regarding seafood consumption for women who are pregnant or breastfeeding and young children. For more information, see the FDA or EPA websites www.FDA.gov/fishadvice; www.EPA.gov/fishadvice.

[e] Assumes food choices to meet food group recommendations are in nutrient-dense forms. Calories from added sugars, solid fats, added refined starches, alcohol, and/or to eat more than the recommended amount of nutrient-dense foods are accounted for under this category.

NOTE: The total eating pattern should not exceed *Dietary Guidelines* limits for intake of calories from added sugars and saturated fats and alcohol and should be within the Acceptable Macronutrient Distribution Ranges for calories from protein, carbohydrate, and total fats. Most calorie patterns do not have enough calories available after meeting food group needs to consume 10 percent of calories from added sugars and 10 percent of calories from saturated fats and still stay within calorie limits. Values are rounded.

Pattern, taking into account food group intakes from studies examining the associations between Mediterranean-Style eating patterns and health.

The Healthy Mediterranean-Style Eating Pattern contains more fruits and seafood and less dairy than does the Healthy U.S.-Style Eating Pattern. The healthfulness of the Healthy Mediterranean-Style Pattern was evaluated based on its similarity to Mediterranean-Style patterns described in studies with positive health outcomes rather than on meeting specified nutrient standards. However, nutrient content of the Pattern was assessed and found to be similar to the Healthy U.S.-Style Eating Pattern, except for calcium and vitamin D. Calcium and vitamin D are lower because the amounts of dairy were decreased, as shown in Appendix 4, to more closely match data from studies of Mediterranean-Style eating patterns.

Healthy Vegetarian Eating Pattern

A Healthy Vegetarian Eating Pattern (Appendix 5) replaces the previous Lacto-ovo Vegetarian Adaptation of the USDA Food Patterns from the *2010 Dietary Guidelines*. The Healthy Vegetarian Eating Pattern was developed taking into account food choices of self-identified vegetarians in the National Health and Nutrition Examination Survey (NHANES) and provides recommendations to meet the *Dietary Guidelines* for those who follow a vegetarian pattern.

In comparison to the Healthy U.S.-Style Eating Pattern, the Healthy Vegetarian Eating Pattern includes more legumes (beans and peas), soy products, nuts and seeds, and whole grains. It contains no meats, poultry, or seafood, and is identical to the Healthy U.S.-Style Eating Pattern in amounts of all other food groups. The Pattern is similar in meeting nutrient standards to the Healthy U.S.-Style Pattern, but is somewhat higher in calcium and dietary fiber and lower in vitamin D, due to differences in the foods included in the protein foods group, specifically more tofu and beans and no seafood, as shown in Appendix 5.

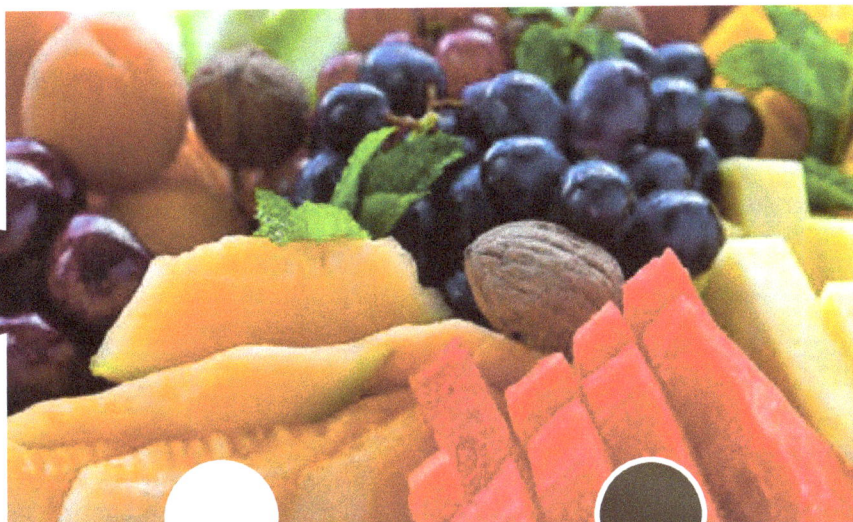

Summary

The *2015-2020 Dietary Guidelines* provides Guidelines and Key Recommendations with clear guidance for individuals to enhance eating and physical activity patterns. Implementation of these Guidelines will help promote health and prevent chronic disease in the United States. At the core of this guidance is the importance of consuming overall healthy eating patterns, including vegetables, fruits, grains, dairy, protein foods, and oils—eaten within an appropriate calorie level and in forms with limited amounts of saturated fats, added sugars, and sodium. Examples of how to put this guidance into practice are provided by the Healthy U.S.-Style Eating Pattern and its two variations, a Healthy Mediterranean-Style Eating Pattern and a Healthy Vegetarian Eating Pattern.

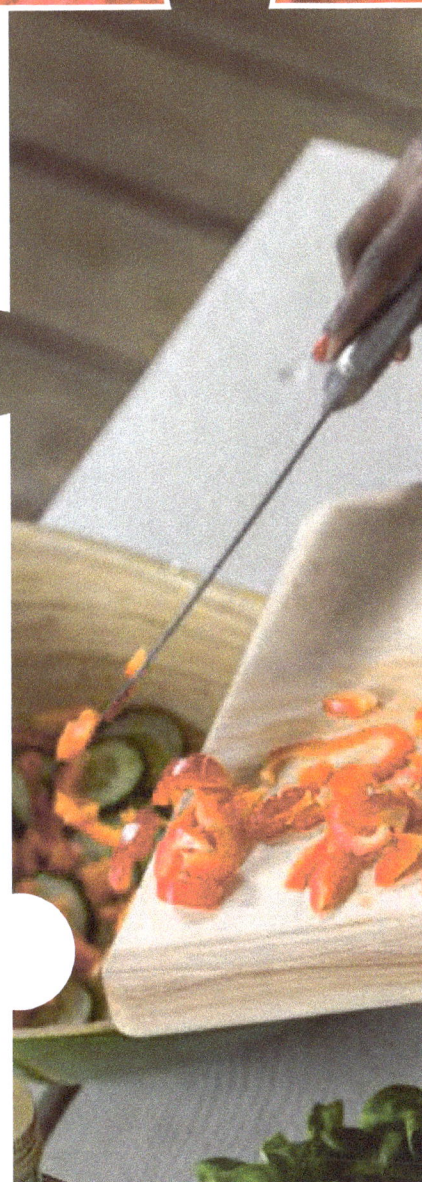

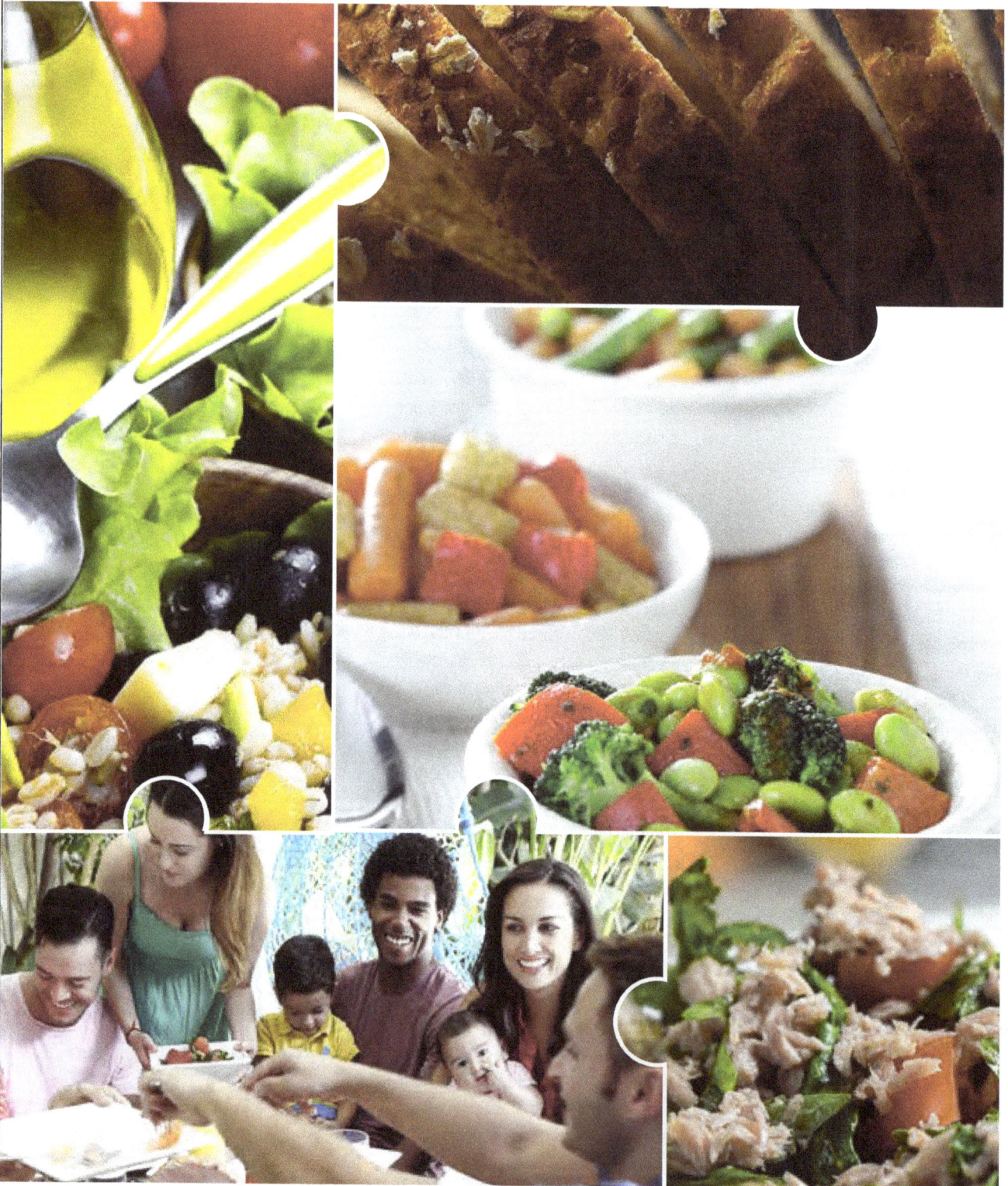

CHAPTER 2
Shifts Needed To Align With Healthy Eating Patterns

Introduction

Following healthy eating patterns is vital to health. This chapter provides a snapshot of current eating patterns of people in the United States in comparison to the recommendations in Chapter 1. Key Elements of Healthy Eating Patterns and describes *shifts* that are needed to align current intakes to recommendations. In some cases, the news is good—for certain aspects of eating patterns, some individuals are following the guidance or are close to meeting the recommendations. However, other aspects of the diet are far from the recommendations. Most Americans would benefit from shifting food choices both within and across food groups and from current food choices to nutrient-dense choices. Some shifts that are needed are minor and can be accomplished by making simple substitutions, while others will require greater effort to accomplish.

About This Chapter

This chapter focuses on the fourth Dietary Guideline:

1. **Follow a healthy eating pattern across the lifespan.** All food and beverage choices matter. Choose a healthy eating pattern at an appropriate calorie level to help achieve and maintain a healthy body weight, support nutrient adequacy, and reduce the risk of chronic disease.

2. **Focus on variety, nutrient density, and amount.** To meet nutrient needs within calorie limits, choose a variety of nutrient-dense foods across and within all food groups in recommended amounts.

3. **Limit calories from added sugars and saturated fats and reduce sodium intake.** Consume an eating pattern low in added sugars, saturated fats, and sodium. Cut back on foods and beverages higher in these components to amounts that fit within healthy eating patterns.

4. ***Shift* to healthier food and beverage choices.** Choose nutrient-dense foods and beverages across and within all food groups in place of less healthy choices. Consider cultural and personal preferences to make these shifts easier to accomplish and maintain.

5. **Support healthy eating patterns for all.** Everyone has a role in helping to create and support healthy eating patterns in multiple settings nationwide, from home to school to work to communities.

The chapter includes quantitative information on intakes and common sources of food groups, their subgroups, and other dietary components, including nutrients. The chapter also includes strategies to help shift current eating patterns toward the healthy patterns described in Chapter 1. Complementary strategies to support individuals in their effort to make shifts are discussed in greater detail in Chapter 3. Everyone Has a Role in Supporting Healthy Eating Patterns.

Current Eating Patterns in the United States

The typical eating patterns currently consumed by many in the United States do not align with the *Dietary Guidelines*. As shown in **Figure 2-1**, when compared to the Healthy U.S.-Style Pattern:

- About three-fourths of the population has an eating pattern that is low in vegetables, fruits, dairy, and oils.

- More than half of the population is meeting or exceeding total grain and total protein foods recommendations, but, as discussed later in the chapter, are not meeting the recommendations for the subgroups within each of these food groups.

- Most Americans exceed the recommendations for added sugars, saturated fats, and sodium.

In addition, the eating patterns of many are too high in calories. Calorie intake over time, in comparison to calorie needs, is best evaluated by measuring body weight status. The high percentage of the population that is overweight or obese suggests that many in the United States overconsume calories. As documented in the **Introduction, Table I-1**, more than two-thirds of all adults and nearly one-third of all children and youth in the United States are either overweight or obese.

Current eating patterns can be moved toward healthier eating patterns by making shifts in food choices over time. Making these shifts can help support a healthy body weight, meet nutrient needs, and lessen the risk for chronic disease.

The following sections highlight average intakes of the food groups and other dietary components for age-sex groups and show that, in some cases, individuals are close to meeting recommendations, but in others, more substantial change is needed. They also provide examples of foods commonly consumed. Understanding what current intakes are and how food groups and other dietary components are consumed can help inform shifts that are needed to support healthy eating patterns.

In this chapter, intakes of food groups and other dietary components are described in two ways:

1. the total amount consumed from all sources in comparison to recommendations or limits, and 2. the proportion of this intake that comes from different food categories based on the form in which foods are eaten—such as soups, sandwiches, or burritos. The What We Eat in American (WWEIA) Food Categories[1] provide insight into the sources of food group and nutrient intakes and are therefore useful in identifying strategies to improve eating patterns.

Figure 2-1.
Dietary Intakes Compared to Recommendations.
Percent of the U.S. Population Ages 1 Year & Older
Who Are Below, At, or Above Each Dietary Goal or Limit

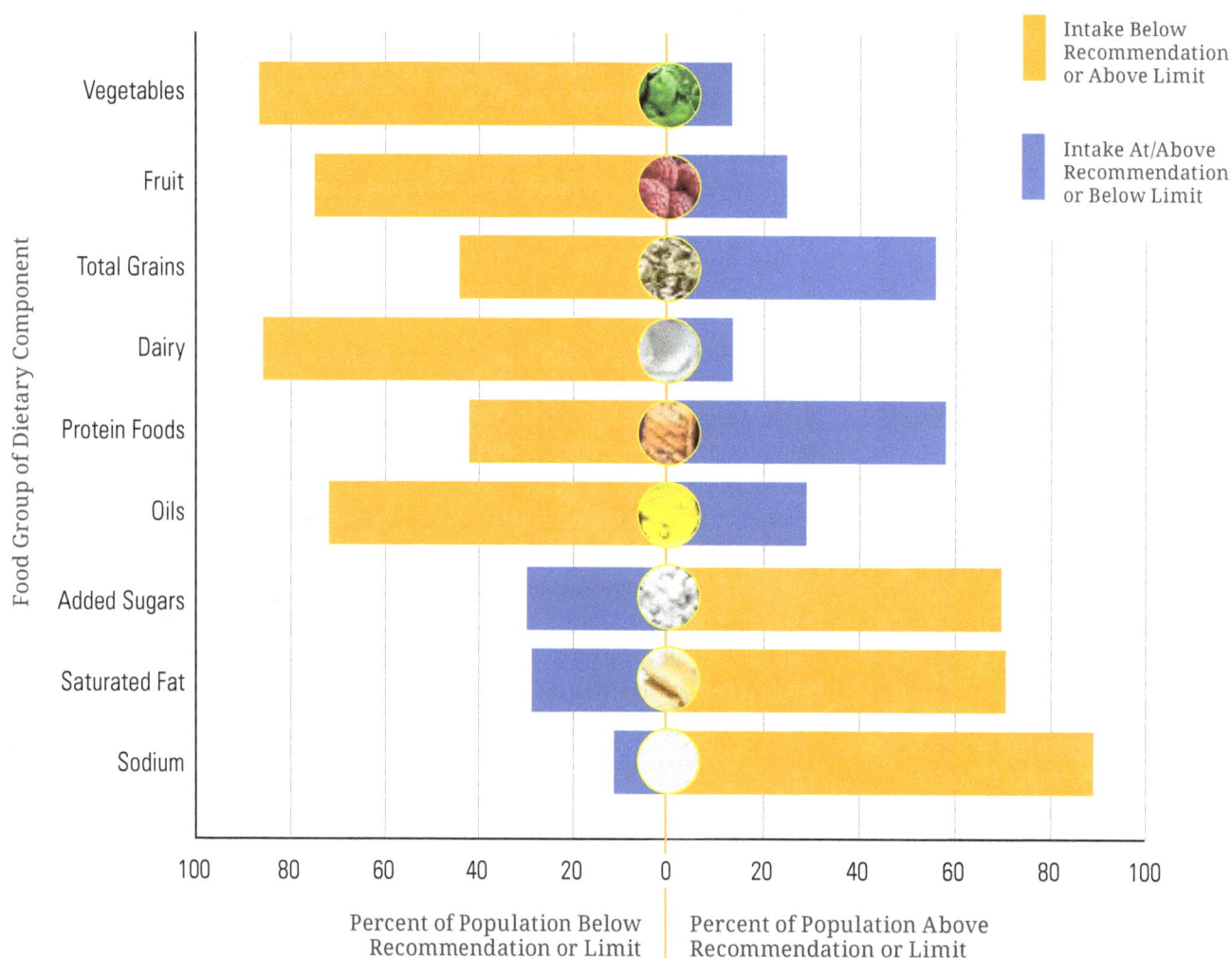

Legend:
- Intake Below Recommendation or Above Limit (orange)
- Intake At/Above Recommendation or Below Limit (blue)

Y-axis (Food Group of Dietary Component): Vegetables, Fruit, Total Grains, Dairy, Protein Foods, Oils, Added Sugars, Saturated Fat, Sodium

X-axis: 100 80 60 40 20 0 20 40 60 80 100

Percent of Population Below Recommendation or Limit | Percent of Population Above Recommendation or Limit

NOTE: The center (0) line is the goal or limit. For most, those represented by the orange sections of the bars, shifting toward the center line will improve their eating pattern.

DATA SOURCES: What We Eat in America, NHANES 2007-2010 for average intakes by age-sex group. Healthy U.S.-Style Food Patterns, which vary based on age, sex, and activity level, for recommended intakes and limits.

[1] The What We Eat in America (WWEIA) Food Categories provide an application to analyze foods and beverages as consumed. Each of the food and beverage items that can be reported in WWEIA, National Health and Nutrition Examination Survey, are placed in one of the mutually exclusive food categories. More information about the WWEIA Food Categories is available at: http://www.ars.usda.gov/Services/docs.htm?docid=23429. Accessed November 25, 2015.

Figure 2-2.
Empower People To Make Healthy Shifts

Making changes to eating patterns can be overwhelming. That's why it's important to emphasize that every food choice is an opportunity to move toward a healthy eating pattern. Small shifts in food choices—over the course of a week, a day, or even a meal—can make a big difference. Here are some ideas for realistic, small shifts that can help people adopt healthy eating patterns.

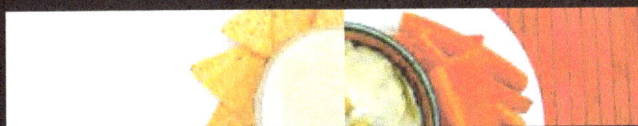

High Calorie Snacks → Nutrient-Dense Snacks

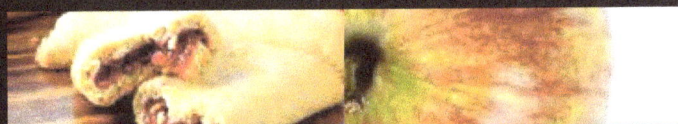

Fruit Products with Added Sugars → Fruit

Refined Grains → Whole Grains

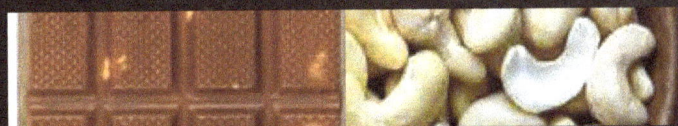

Snacks with Added Sugars → Unsalted Snacks

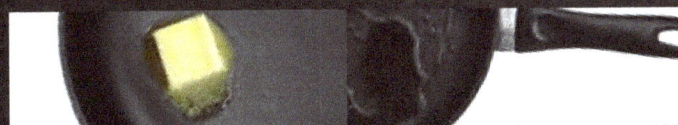

Solid Fats → Oils

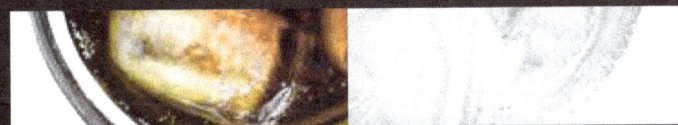

Beverages with Added Sugars → No-Sugar-Added Beverages

Changing Physical Activity Patterns for a Healthy Lifestyle

Current Physical Activity:
Only 20 percent of adults meet the Physical Activity Guidelines for aerobic and muscle-strengthening activity. Males are more likely to report doing regular physical activity compared to females (24% of males versus 17% of females meet recommendations), and this difference is more pronounced between adolescent boys and girls (30% of males versus 13% of females meet recommendations). Despite evidence that increments of physical activity as short as 10 minutes at a time can be beneficial, about 30 percent of adults report engaging in no leisure time physical activity. Disparities also exist; individuals with lower income and those with lower educational attainment have lower rates of physical activity and are more likely to not engage in leisure time physical activity.

Overall, physical activity associated with work, home, and transportation has declined in recent decades and can be attributed to less active occupations; reduced physical activity for commuting to work, school, or for errands; and increased sedentary behavior often associated with television viewing and other forms of screen time.

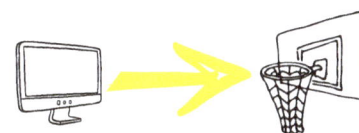

***Shift* Physical Activity Choices:**
Most individuals would benefit from making shifts to increase the amount of physical activity they engage in each week. Individuals would also benefit from limiting screen time and decreasing the amount of time spent being sedentary.

Figure 2-3.

Average Daily Food Group Intakes by Age-Sex Groups, Compared to Ranges of Recommended Intake

■ Recommended Intake Ranges
◯ Average Intake

Vegetables

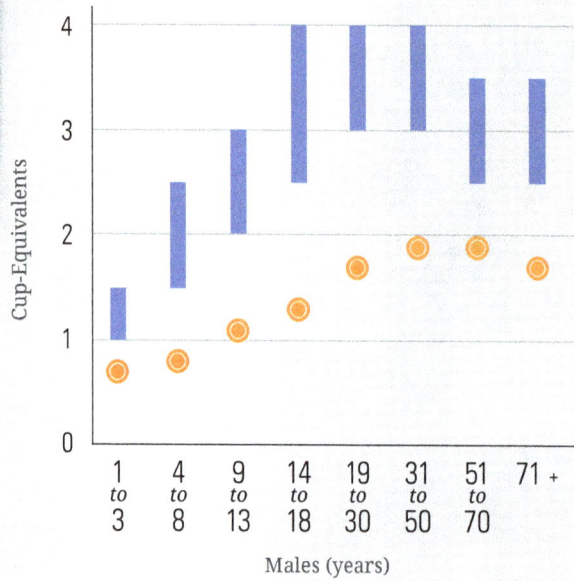

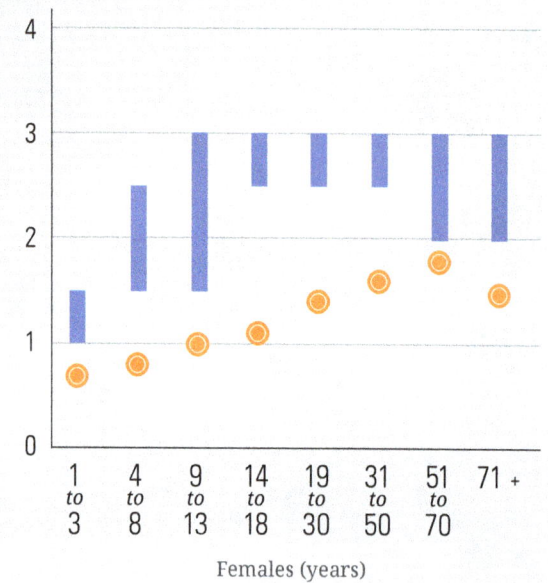

Fruits

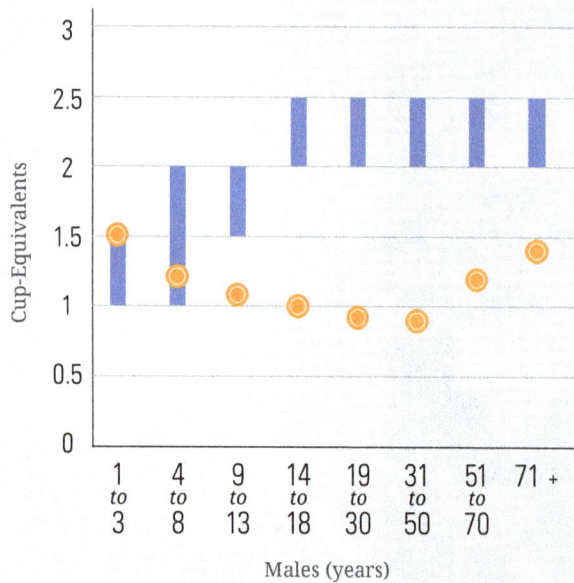

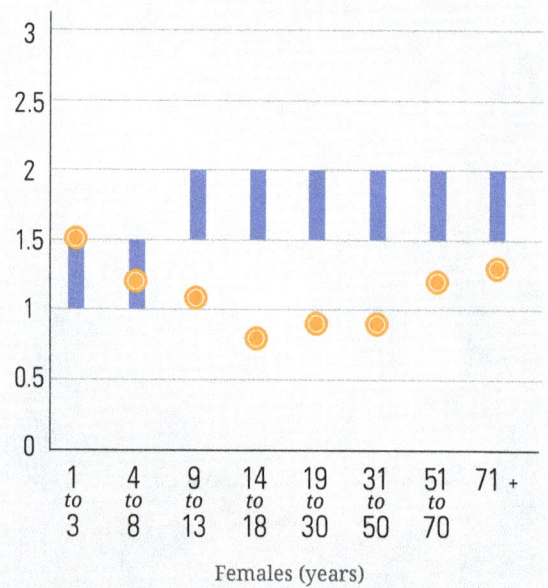

Recommended Intake Ranges ■   **Average Intake** ⬤

Total Grains

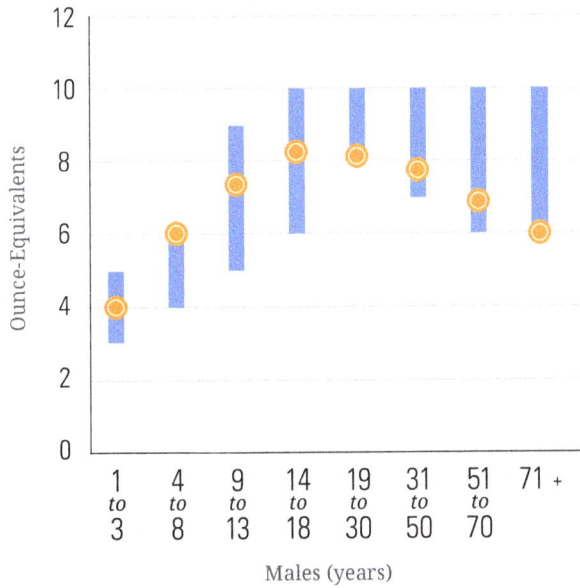

Males (years)

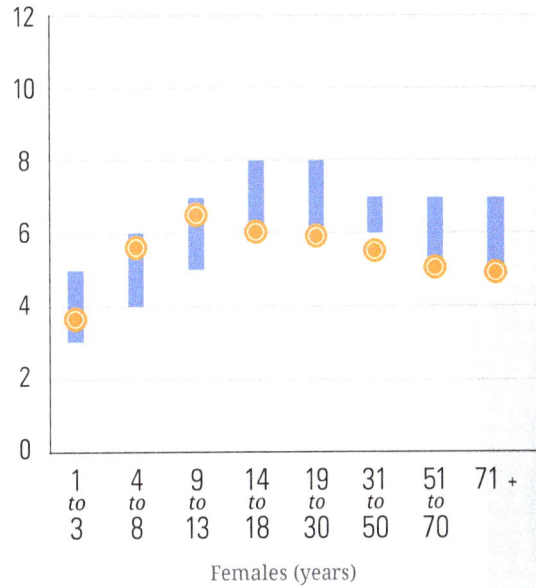

Females (years)

Dairy

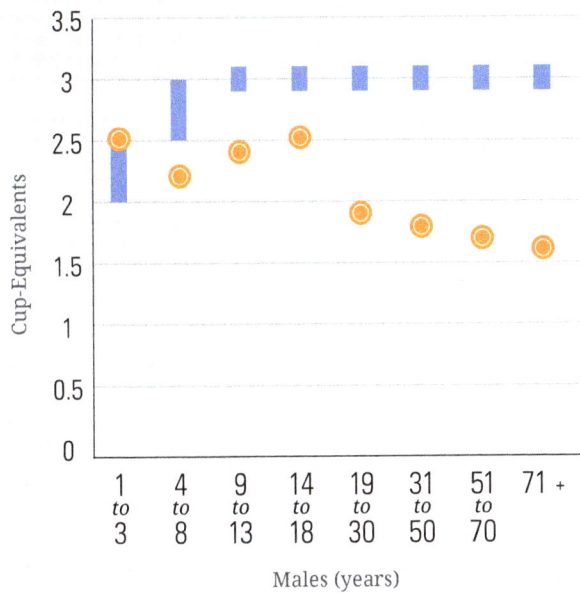

Males (years)

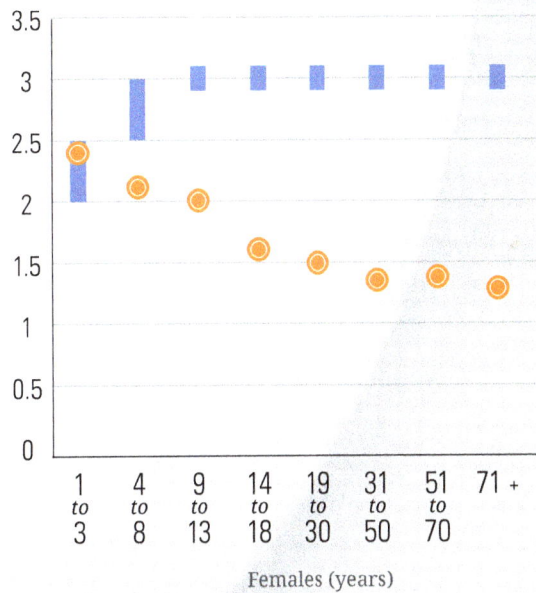

Females (years)

Figure 2-3. *(continued...)*

Average Daily Food Group Intakes by Age-Sex Groups, Compared to Ranges of Recommended Intake

■ Recommended Intake Ranges
○ Average Intake

Protein Foods

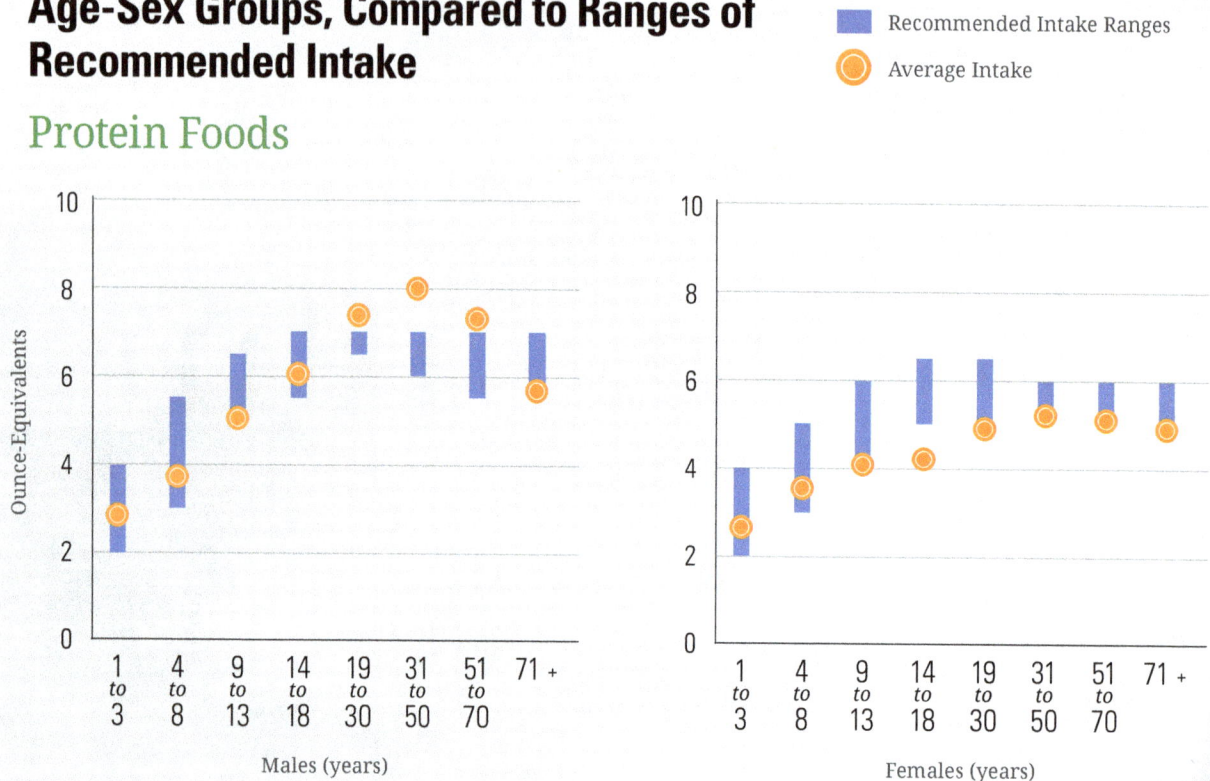

Males (years)

Females (years)

DATA SOURCES: What We Eat in America, NHANES 2007-2010 for average intakes by age-sex group. Healthy U.S.-Style Food Patterns, which vary based on age, sex, and activity level, for recommended intake ranges.

A Closer Look at Current Intakes & Recommended Shifts

As described in Chapter 1, most foods in healthy eating patterns should come from the food groups. As **Figure 2-3** shows, across the U.S. population, average intakes of foods from the food groups are far from amounts recommended in the Healthy U.S.-Style Eating Pattern.

Food Groups

The following sections describe total current intakes for each of the food groups and for oils, and the leading food categories contributing to this total. They also describe the shifts in food choices that are needed to meet recommendations and provide strategies that can help individuals make these shifts.

Vegetables

Current Intakes: Figure 2-3 shows the low average intakes of vegetables across age-sex groups in comparison to recommended intake levels. Vegetable consumption relative to recommendations is lowest among boys ages 9 to 13 years and girls ages 14 to 18 years. Vegetable intakes relative to recommendations are slightly higher during the adult years, but intakes are still below recommendations. In addition, with few exceptions, the U.S. population does not meet intake recommendations for any of the vegetable subgroups (**Figure 2-4**).

Calories in Nutrient-Dense Versus Current Typical Choices in the Food Groups

To stay within energy requirements while meeting nutritional needs, food choices in each food group should be in nutrient-dense forms. However, in many food groups, foods as they are typically eaten are not in nutrient-dense forms—they contain additional calories from components such as added sugars, added refined starches, solid fats, or a combination. For example, in the dairy group, nutrient-dense choices such as fat-free milk, plain fat-free yogurt, and low-fat cheese contain an average of about 80 calories per cup-equivalent. In contrast, many dairy products that are typically consumed, such as whole milk, sweetened yogurt, and regular cheese, contain almost 150 calories per cup-equivalent.[2] Similarly, in the protein foods group, nutrient-dense (lean) choices of meats and poultry contain an average of about 50 calories per ounce-equivalent, but the higher fat choices that are typically consumed contain about 80 to 100 calories per ounce-equivalent. Grains and vegetables also are often consumed in forms that contain additional calories from added sugars or solid fats that are added in processing or preparing the food, rather than in nutrient-dense forms.

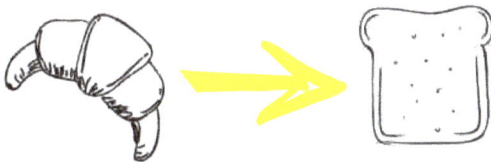

When typical instead of nutrient-dense choices are made in each food group, individuals consume extra calories when meeting their food group recommendations. Shifting from typical choices to nutrient-dense options is an important principle for maintaining calorie balance in a healthy eating pattern. A related principle, reducing the portion size of foods and beverages that are not in nutrient-dense forms, also can help to maintain calorie balance.

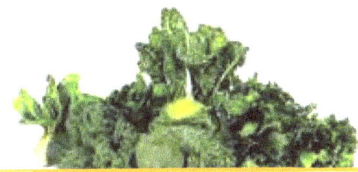

Figure 2-4.

Average Vegetable Subgroup Intakes in Cup-Equivalents per Week by Age-Sex Groups, Compared to Ranges of Recommended Intakes per Week

Dark Green Vegetables

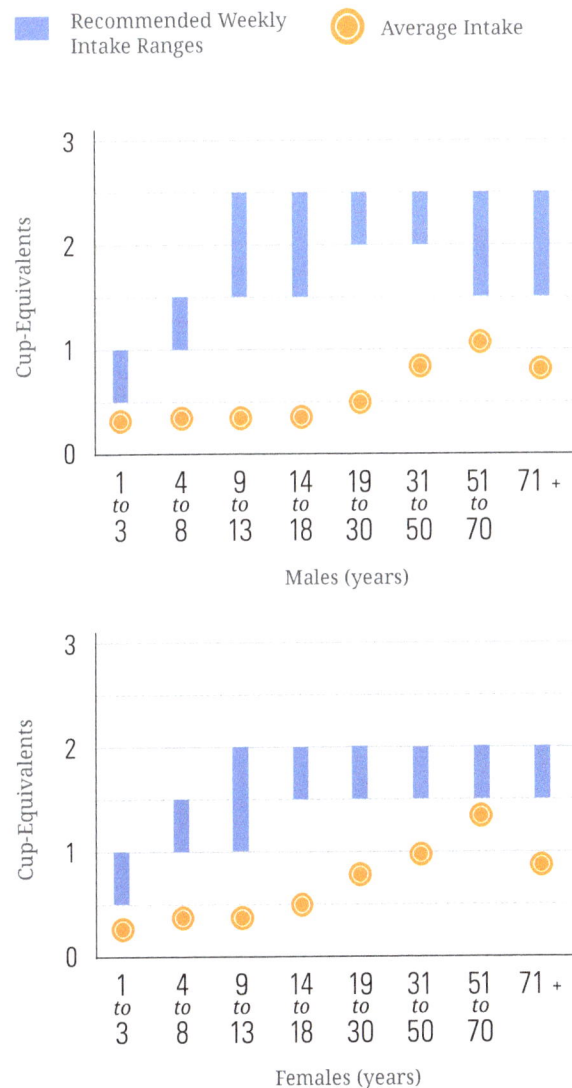

[2] Britten P, Cleveland LE, Koegel KL, Kuczynski KJ, and Nickols-Richardson MS. Impact of typical rather than nutrient dense food choices in the US Department of Agriculture Food Patterns. *J Acad Nutr Diet.* 2012;112 (10):1560-1569.

Figure 2-4. *(continued...)*
Average Vegetable Subgroup Intakes in Cup-Equivalents per Week by Age-Sex Groups, Compared to Ranges of Recommended Intakes per Week

■ Recommended Intake Range
○ Average Intake

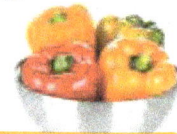

Red & Orange Vegetables

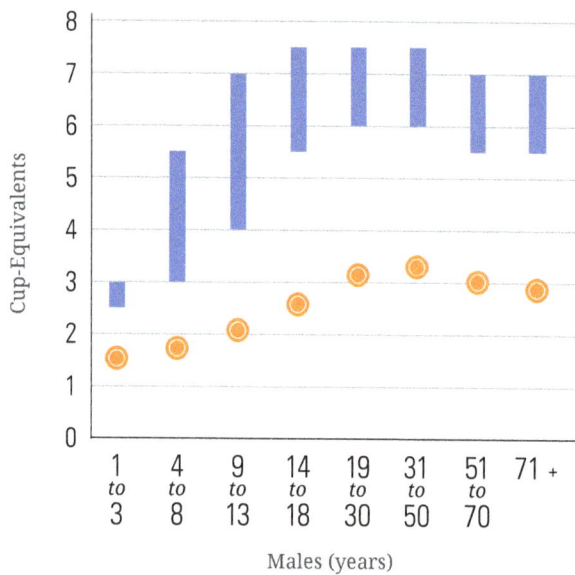

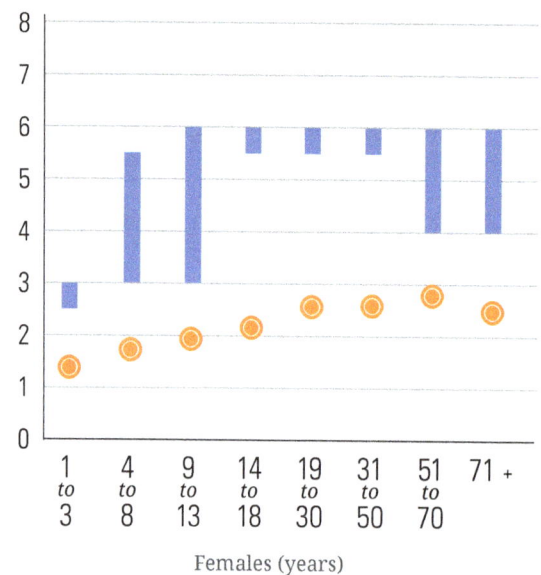

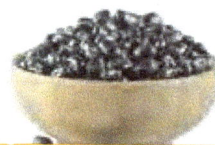

Males (years)

Females (years)

Legumes (Beans & Peas)

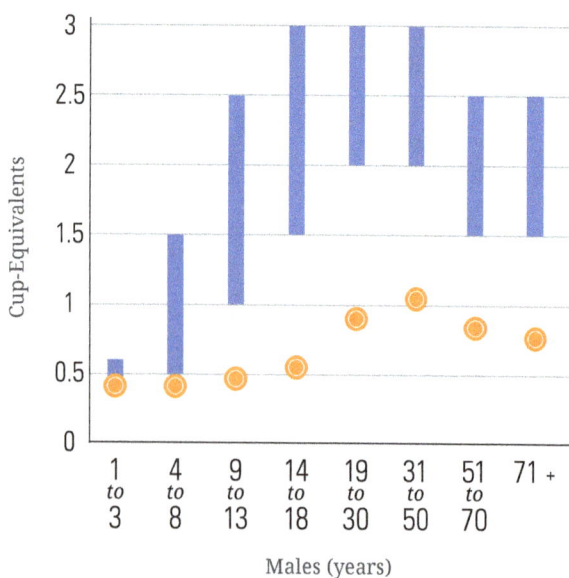

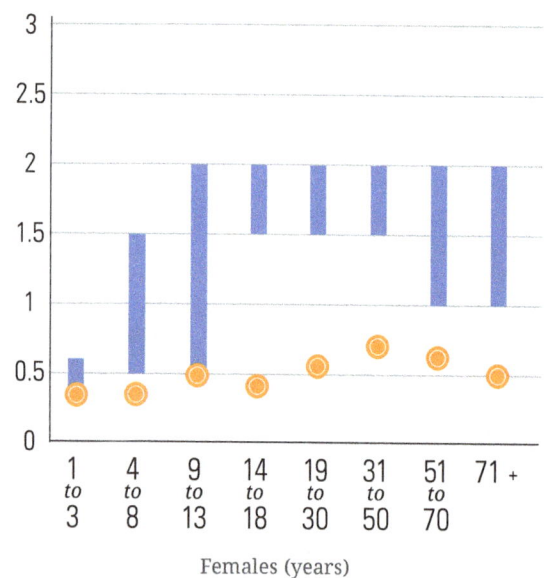

Males (years)

Females (years)

■ Recommended Intake Ranges ◉ Average Intake

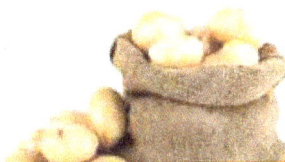

Starchy Vegetables

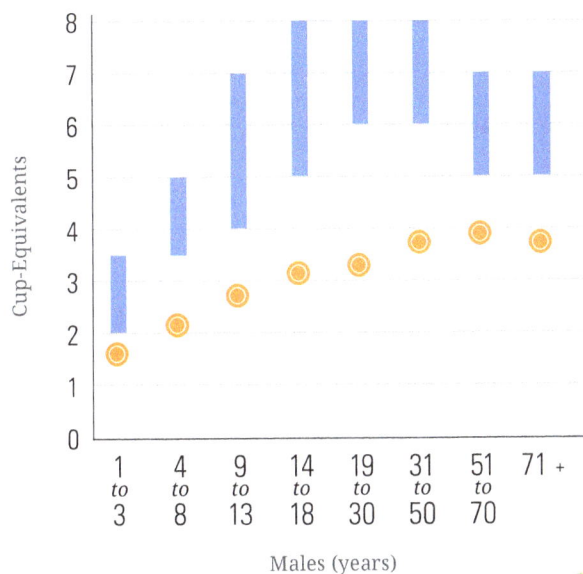

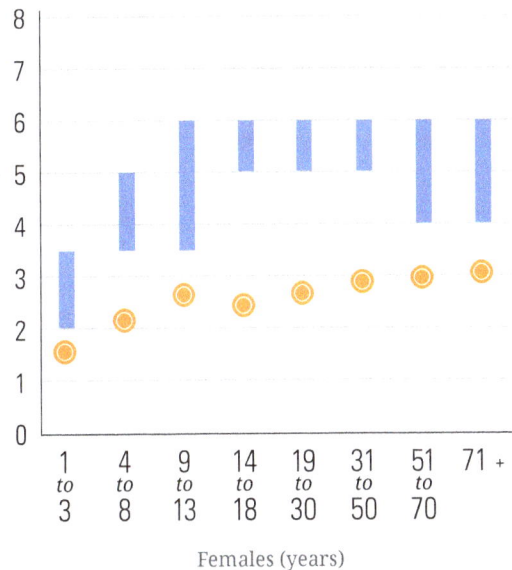

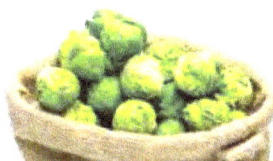

Cup-Equivalents

| 1 to 3 | 4 to 8 | 9 to 13 | 14 to 18 | 19 to 30 | 31 to 50 | 51 to 70 | 71 + |

Males (years)

Females (years)

Other Vegetables

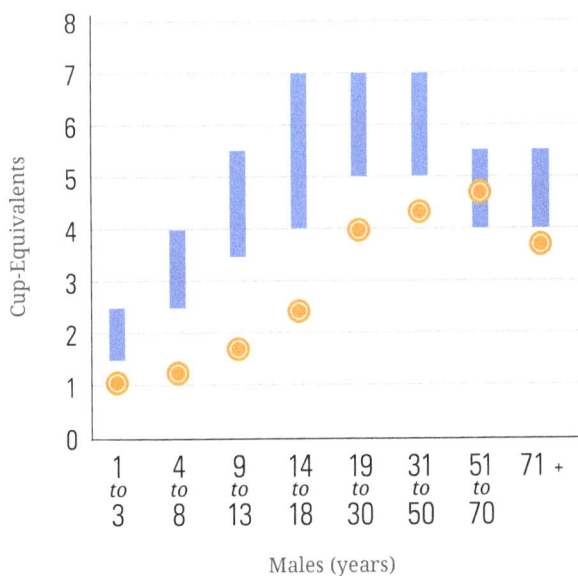

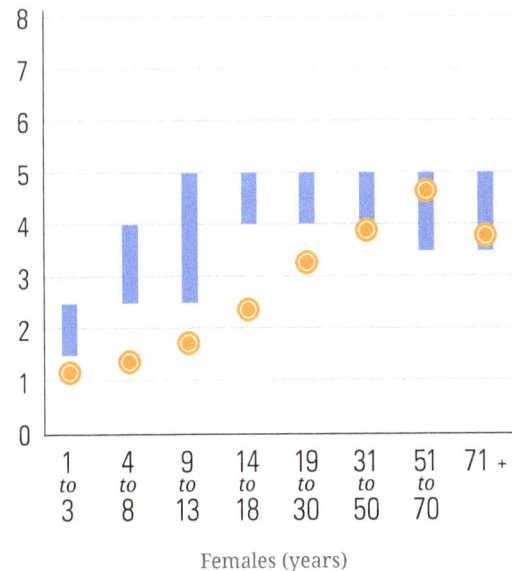

Cup-Equivalents

| 1 to 3 | 4 to 8 | 9 to 13 | 14 to 18 | 19 to 30 | 31 to 50 | 51 to 70 | 71 + |

Males (years)

Females (years)

DATA SOURCES: What We Eat in America, NHANES 2007-2010 for average intakes by age-sex group. Healthy U.S.-Style Food Patterns, which vary based on age, sex, and activity level, for recommended intake ranges.

Potatoes and tomatoes are the most commonly consumed vegetables, accounting for 21 percent and 18 percent of all vegetable consumption, respectively. Lettuce and onions are the only other vegetables that make up more than 5 percent each of total vegetable group consumption. **Table 2-1** lists additional examples of vegetables in each of the subgroups. About 60 percent of all vegetables are eaten as a separate food item, about 30 percent as part of a mixed dish, and the remaining 10 percent as part of snack foods, condiments, and gravies. Vegetables are part of many types of mixed dishes, from burgers, sandwiches, and tacos to pizza, meat stews, pasta dishes, grain-based casseroles, and soups.

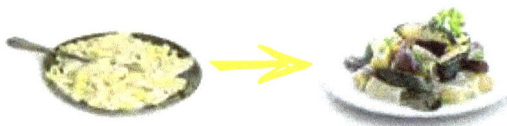

Shift **To Consume More Vegetables:**

For most individuals, following a healthy eating pattern would include an increase in total vegetable intake from all vegetable subgroups, in nutrient-dense forms, and an increase in the variety of different vegetables consumed over time (see **Table 2-1**). Strategies to increase vegetable intake include choosing more vegetables—from all subgroups—in place of foods high in calories, saturated fats, or sodium such as some meats, poultry, cheeses, and snack foods. One realistic option is to increase the vegetable content of mixed dishes while decreasing the amounts of other food components that are often overconsumed, such as refined grains or meats high in saturated fat and/or sodium. Other strategies include always choosing a green salad or a vegetable as a side dish and incorporating vegetables into most meals and snacks.

Table 2-1.

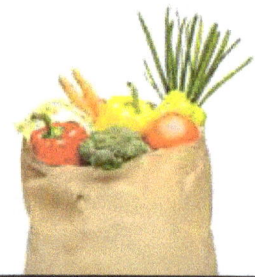

Examples of Vegetables in Each Vegetable Subgroup

Vegetable Subgroup	Examples
Dark-Green Vegetables	Broccoli, Spinach, Leafy Salad Greens (Including Romaine Lettuce), Collards, Bok Choy, Kale, Turnip Greens, Mustard Greens, Green Herbs (Parsley, Cilantro)
Red & Orange Vegetables	Tomatoes, Carrots, Tomato Juice, Sweet Potatoes, Red Peppers (Hot and Sweet), Winter Squash, Pumpkin
Legumes (Beans & Peas)	Pinto, White, Kidney, and Black Beans; Lentils; Chickpeas; Limas (Mature, Dried); Split Peas; Edamame (Green Soybeans)
Starchy Vegetables	Potatoes, Corn, Green Peas, Limas (Green, Immature), Plantains, Cassava
Other Vegetables	Lettuce (Iceberg), Onions, Green Beans, Cucumbers, Celery, Green Peppers, Cabbage, Mushrooms, Avocado, Summer Squash (Includes Zucchini), Cauliflower, Eggplant, Garlic, Bean Sprouts, Olives, Asparagus, Peapods (Snowpeas), Beets

Fruits

Current Intakes: As shown in **Figure 2-3**, average intake of fruits is below recommendations for almost all age-sex groups. Children ages 1 to 8 years differ from the rest of the population in that many do meet recommended intakes for total fruit. Average intakes of fruits, including juice, are lowest among girls ages 14 to 18 years and adults ages 19 to 50 years. Older women (ages 51 years and older) and young children consume fruits in amounts close to or meeting minimum recommended intakes (**Figure 2-3**).

About one-third of the intake of fruits in the U.S. population comes from fruit juice, and the remaining two-thirds from whole fruits (which includes cut up, cooked, canned, frozen, and dried fruits). The highest proportion of juice to whole fruits intake is among children ages 1 to 3 years, for whom about 47 percent of total fruit intake comes from fruit juice, and about 53 percent from whole fruits. Average juice intakes for young children are within the limits recommended by the American Academy of Pediatrics (see the Fruits section of Chapter 1).

Fruits and fruit juices are most likely to be consumed alone or in a mixture with other fruit, rather than as part of a mixed dish that includes foods from other food groups. Almost 90 percent of all fruit intake comes from single fruits, fruit salads, or fruit juices. The most commonly consumed fruits are apples, bananas, watermelon, grapes, strawberries, oranges, peaches, cantaloupe, pears, blueberries, raisins, and pineapple. Commonly consumed fruit juices are orange juice, apple juice, and grape juice.

Figure 2-5.

Average Whole & Refined Grain Intakes in Ounce-Equivalents per Day by Age-Sex Groups, Compared to Ranges of Recommended Daily Intake for Whole Grains & Limits for Refined Grains*

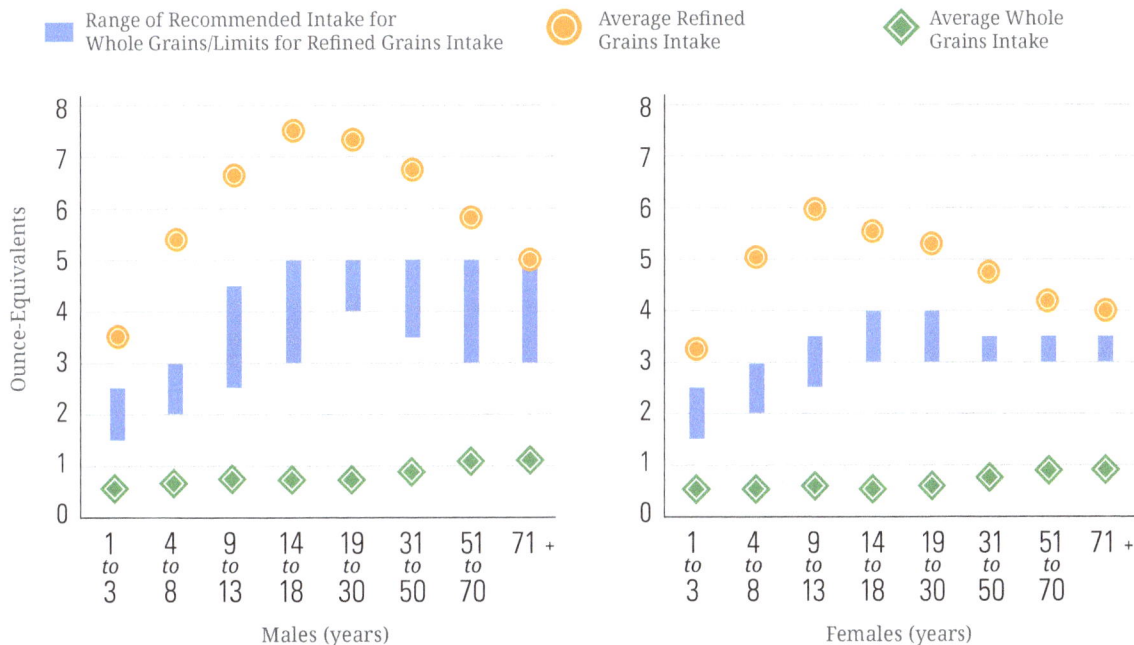

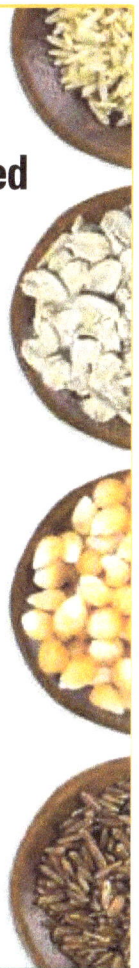

■ Range of Recommended Intake for Whole Grains/Limits for Refined Grains Intake   ⬤ Average Refined Grains Intake   ◆ Average Whole Grains Intake

Males (years): 1 to 3, 4 to 8, 9 to 13, 14 to 18, 19 to 30, 31 to 50, 51 to 70, 71+

Females (years): 1 to 3, 4 to 8, 9 to 13, 14 to 18, 19 to 30, 31 to 50, 51 to 70, 71+

Ounce-Equivalents

*NOTE: Recommended daily intake of whole grains is to be at least half of total grain consumption, and the limit for refined grains is to be no more than half of total grain consumption. The blue vertical bars on this graph represent one half of the total grain recommendations for each age-sex group, and therefore indicate recommendations for the minimum amounts to consume of whole grains or maximum amounts of refined grains. To meet recommendations, whole grain intake should be within or above the blue bars and refined grain intake within or below the bars.

DATA SOURCES: What We Eat in America, NHANES 2007-2010 for average intakes by age-sex group. Healthy U.S.-Style Food Patterns, which vary based on age, sex, and activity level, for recommended intake ranges.

***Shift* To Consume More Fruits:**

To help support healthy eating patterns, most individuals in the United States would benefit from increasing their intake of fruits, mostly whole fruits, in nutrient-dense forms. A wide variety of fruits are available in the U.S. marketplace, some year-round and others seasonally. Strategies to help achieve this shift include choosing more fruits as snacks, in salads, as side dishes, and as desserts in place of foods with added sugars, such as cakes, pies, cookies, doughnuts, ice cream, and candies.

Grains

Current Intakes: Intakes of total grains are close to the target amounts (**Figure 2-3**) for all age-sex groups, but as shown in **Figure 2-5**, intakes do not meet the recommendations for whole grains and exceed limits for refined grains. Average intakes of whole grains are far below recommended levels across all age-sex groups, and average intakes of refined grains are well above recommended limits for most age-sex groups.

Examples of commonly consumed whole-grain foods are whole-wheat breads, rolls, bagels, and crackers; oatmeal; whole-grain ready-to-eat cereals (e.g., shredded wheat, oat rings); popcorn; brown rice; and whole-grain pasta. Examples of refined grain foods are white bread, rolls, bagels, and crackers; pasta; pizza crust; grain based desserts; refined grain ready-to-eat cereals (e.g., corn flakes, crispy rice cereal); corn and wheat tortillas; white rice; and cornbread. As noted in Chapter 1, most refined grain foods in the United States are made from enriched grains. Almost half of all refined grains intake is from mixed dishes, such as burgers, sandwiches, tacos, pizza, macaroni and cheese, and spaghetti with meatballs. About 20 percent of refined grain intake comes from snacks and sweets, including cakes, cookies, and other grain desserts. The remaining 30 percent of refined grain intake is eaten as a separate food item, such as cereals, breads, or rice. About 60 percent of whole-grain intake in the United States is from individual food items, mostly cereals, rather than mixed dishes.

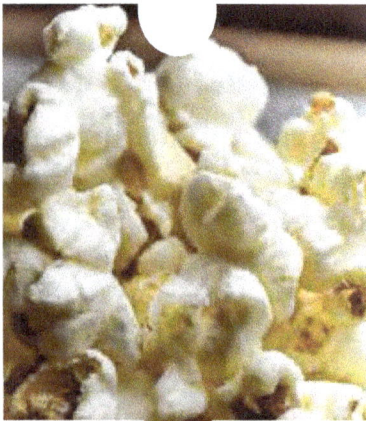

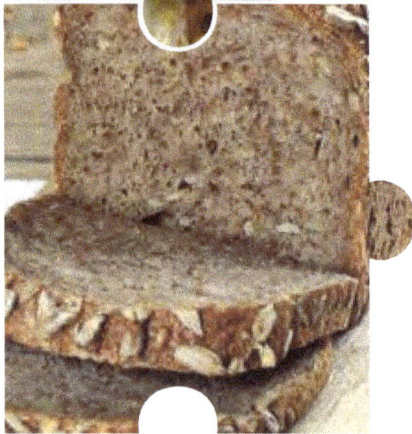

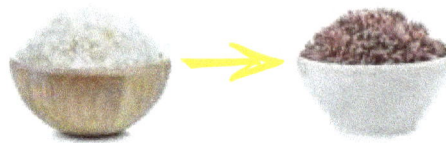

Shift To Make Half of All Grains Consumed Be Whole Grains:

Shifting from refined to whole-grain versions of commonly consumed foods—such as from white to 100% whole-wheat breads, white to whole-grain pasta, and white to brown rice—would increase whole-grain intakes and lower refined grain intakes to help meet recommendations. Strategies to increase whole grains in place of refined grains include using the ingredient list on packaged foods to select foods that have whole grains listed as the first grain ingredient. Another strategy is to cut back on refined grain desserts and sweet snacks such as cakes, cookies, and pastries, which are high in added sugars, solid fats, or both, and are a common source of excess calories. Choosing both whole and refined grain foods in nutrient-dense forms, such as choosing plain popcorn instead of buttered, bread instead of croissants, and English muffins instead of biscuits also can help in meeting recommendations for a healthy eating pattern.

Dairy

Current Intakes: As shown in **Figure 2-3**, average intakes of dairy for most age-sex groups are far below recommendations of the Healthy U.S.-Style Pattern. Average dairy intake for most young children ages 1 to 3 years meets recommended amounts, but all other age groups have average intakes that are below recommendations. An

age-related decline in dairy intake begins in childhood, and intakes persist at low levels for adults of all ages.

Fluid milk (51%) and cheese (45%) comprise most of dairy consumption. Yogurt (2.6%) and fortified soy beverages (commonly known as "soymilk") (1.5%) make up the rest of dairy intake. About three-fourths of all milk is consumed as a beverage or on cereal, but cheese is most commonly consumed as part of mixed dishes, such as burgers, sandwiches, tacos, pizza, and pasta dishes.

Shift To Consume More Dairy Products in Nutrient-Dense Forms:

Most individuals in the United States would benefit by increasing dairy intake in fat-free or low-fat forms, whether from milk (including lactose-free milk), yogurt, and cheese or from fortified soy beverages (soymilk). Some sweetened milk and yogurt products may be included in a healthy eating pattern as long as the total amount of added sugars consumed does not exceed the limit for added sugars, and the eating pattern does not exceed calorie limits. Because most cheese contains more sodium and saturated fats, and less potassium, vitamin A, and vitamin D than milk or yogurt, increased intake of dairy products would be most beneficial if more fat-free or low-fat milk and yogurt were selected rather than cheese. Strategies to increase dairy intake include drinking fat-free or low-fat milk (or a fortified soy beverage) with meals, choosing yogurt as a snack, or using yogurt as an ingredient in prepared dishes such as salad dressings or spreads. Strategies for choosing dairy products in nutrient-dense forms include choosing lower fat versions of milk, yogurt, and cheese in place of whole milk products and regular cheese.

Protein Foods

Current Intakes: Overall, average intakes of protein foods are close to amounts recommended for all age-sex groups (**Figure 2-3**). However, **Figure 2-6** shows that the average intakes of protein foods subgroups vary in comparison to the range of intake recommendations. Overall, average intakes of seafood are low for all age-sex groups; average intakes of nuts, seeds, and soy products are close to recommended levels; and

average intakes of meats, poultry, and eggs are high for teen boys and adult men. Legumes (beans and peas), a vegetables subgroup, also may be considered as part of the protein foods group (see the About Legumes (Beans and Peas) call-out box in Chapter 1). As shown in **Figure 2-4**, intakes of legumes are below vegetable group recommendations.

Commonly consumed protein foods include beef (especially ground beef), chicken, pork, processed meats (e.g., hot dogs,

sausages, ham, luncheon meats), and eggs. The most common seafood choices are shrimp, tuna, and salmon; and the most common nut choices are peanuts, peanut butter, almonds, and mixed nuts. Slightly less than half (49%) of all protein foods are consumed as a separate food item, such as a chicken breast, a steak, an egg, a fish filet, or peanuts. About the same proportion are consumed as part of a mixed dish (45%), with the largest amount from burgers, sandwiches, and tacos.

Figure 2-6.

Average Protein Foods Subgroup Intakes in Ounce-Equivalents per Week by Age-Sex Groups, Compared to Ranges of Recommended Intake

Meats, Poultry, & Eggs

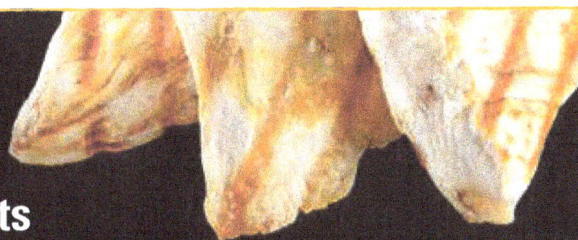

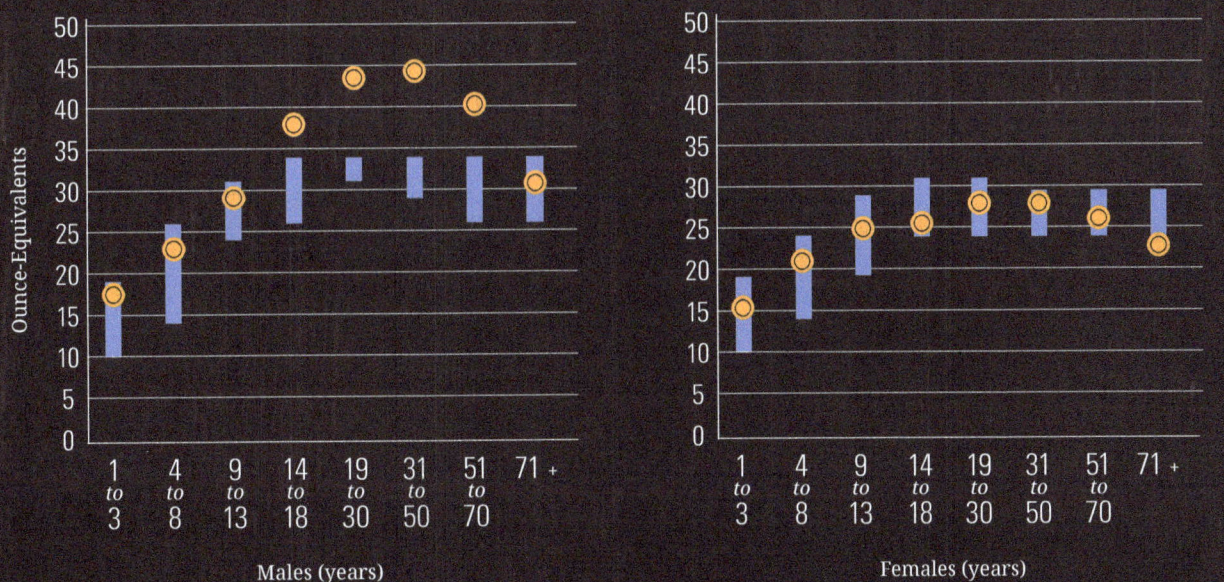

Figure 2-6. *(continued...)*

Average Protein Foods Subgroup Intakes in Ounce-Equivalents per Week by Age-Sex Groups, Compared to Ranges of Recommended Intake

■ Recommended Weekly Intake Ranges

◉ Average Weekly Intake

Seafood

Males (years)

Females (years)

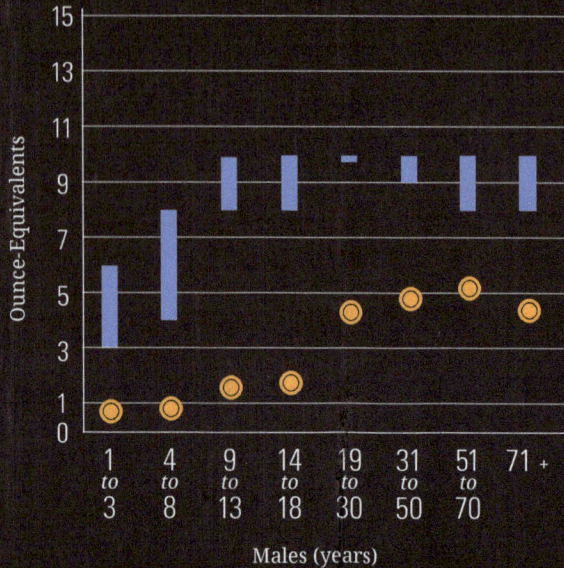

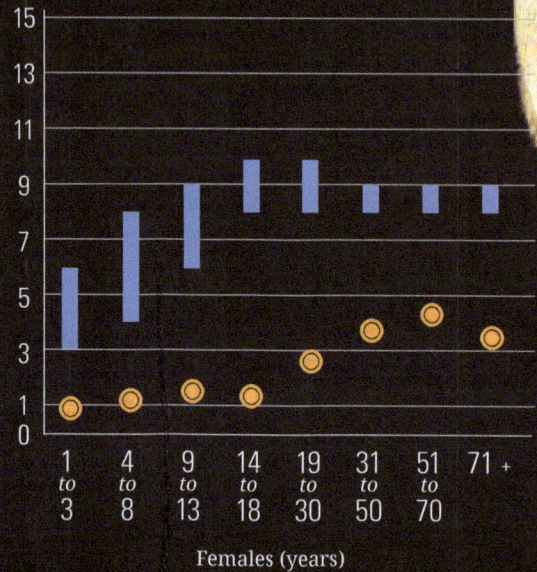

Nuts, Seeds, & Soy Products

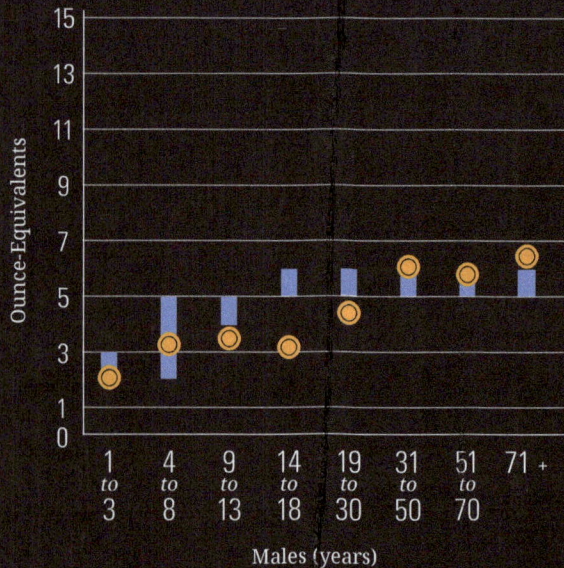

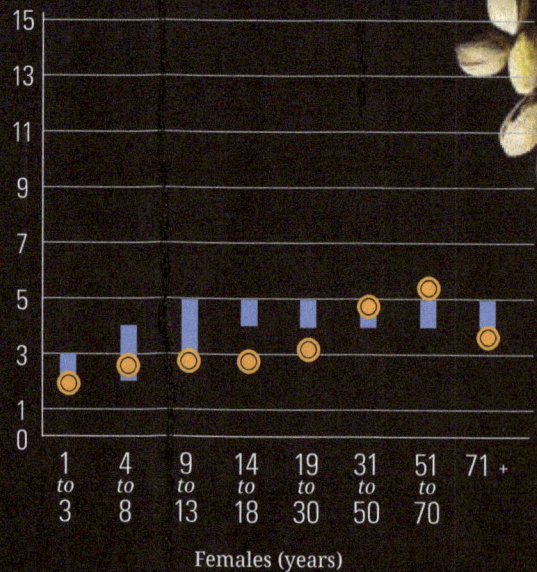

Males (years)

Females (years)

DATA SOURCES: What We Eat in America, NHANES 2007-2010 for average intakes by age-sex group. Healthy U.S.-Style Food Patterns, which vary based on age, sex, and activity level, for recommended intake ranges.

Average intake of total protein foods is close to recommendations, while average seafood intake is below recommendations for all age-sex groups. Shifts are needed within the protein foods group to increase seafood intake, but the foods to be replaced depend on the individual's current intake from the other protein subgroups. Strategies to increase the variety of protein foods include incorporating seafood as the protein foods choice in meals twice per week in place of meat, poultry, or eggs, and using legumes or nuts and seeds in mixed dishes instead of some meat or poultry. For example, choosing a salmon steak, a tuna sandwich, bean chili, or almonds on a main-dish salad could all increase protein variety.

Shifting to nutrient-dense options, including lean and lower sodium options, will improve the nutritional quality of protein food choices and support healthy eating patterns. Some individuals, especially teen boys and adult men, also need to reduce overall intake of protein foods (see **Figure 2-3**) by decreasing intakes of meats, poultry, and eggs and increasing amounts of vegetables or other underconsumed food groups.

Oils

Current Intakes: Average intakes of oils are below the recommendations for almost every age-sex group (**Figure 2-7**). However, intakes are not far from recommendations. In the United States, most oils are consumed in packaged foods, such as salad dressings, mayonnaise,

Figure 2-7.

Average Intakes of Oils & Solid Fats in Grams per Day by Age-Sex Group, in Comparison to Ranges of Recommended Intake for Oils

Legend:
- ■ Recommended Oils Intake Range
- ● Average Solid Fats Intake
- ◆ Average Oils Intake

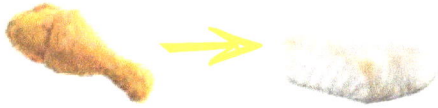

Males (years): 1 to 3, 4 to 8, 9 to 13, 14 to 18, 19 to 30, 31 to 50, 51 to 70, 71 +

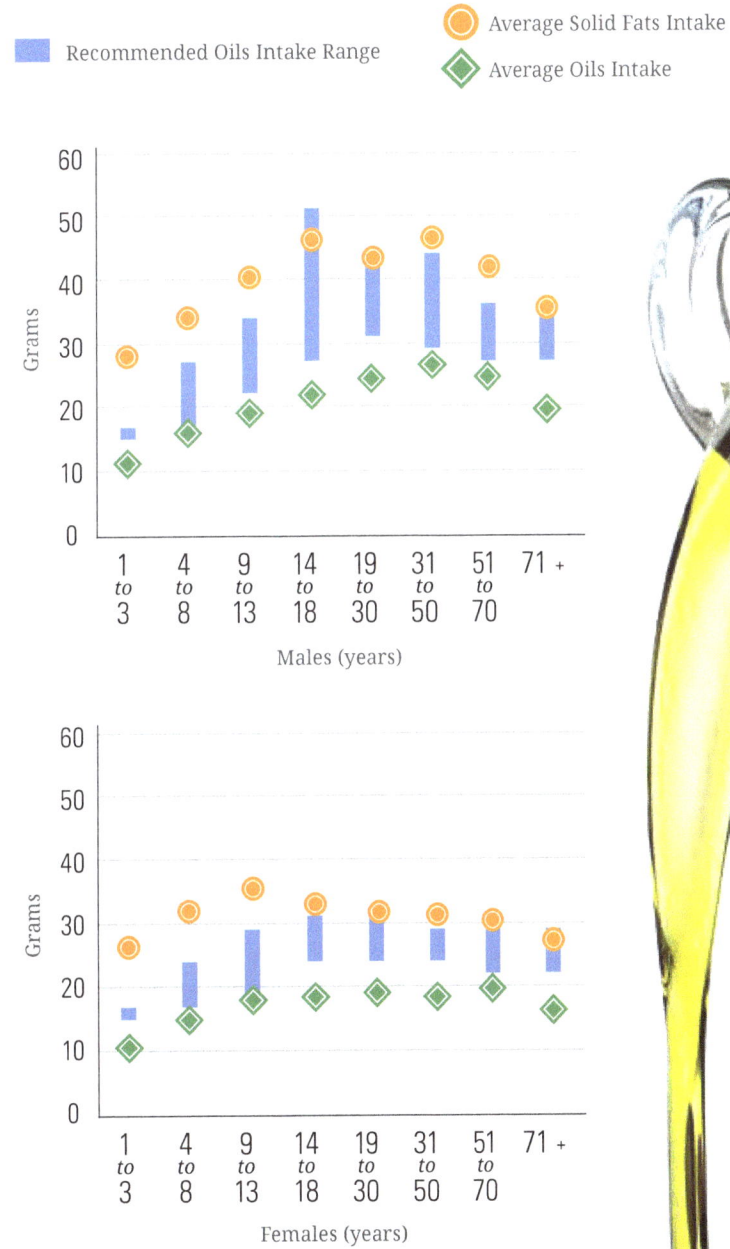

Females (years): 1 to 3, 4 to 8, 9 to 13, 14 to 18, 19 to 30, 31 to 50, 51 to 70, 71 +

DATA SOURCES: What We Eat in America, NHANES 2007-2010 for average intakes by age-sex group. Healthy U.S. Style Food Patterns, which vary based on age, sex, and activity level, for recommended intake ranges.

prepared vegetables, snack chips (corn and potato), and as part of nuts and seeds. Oils also can be used in preparing foods such as stir-fries and sautés. The most commonly used oil in the United States is soybean oil. Other commonly used oils include canola, corn, olive, cottonseed, sunflower, and peanut oil. Oils also are found in nuts, avocados, and seafood. Coconut, palm, and palm kernel oils (tropical oils) are solid at room temperature because they have high amounts of saturated fatty acids and are therefore classified as a solid fat rather than as an oil. (See Chapter 1 for more information on tropical oils.)

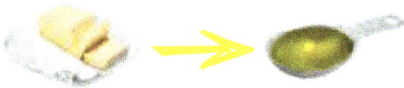

Shift From Solid Fats to Oils:

To move the intake of oils to recommended levels, individuals should use oils rather than solid fats in food preparation where possible. Strategies to shift intake include using vegetable oil in place of solid fats (butter, stick margarine, shortening, lard, coconut oil) when cooking, increasing the intake of foods that naturally contain oils, such as seafood and nuts, in place of some meat and poultry, and choosing other foods, such as salad dressings and spreads, made with oils instead of solid fats.

Other Dietary Components

As described in Chapter 1, in addition to the food groups, other components also should be considered when building healthy eating patterns, including limiting the amounts of added sugars, saturated fats, and sodium consumed. Additionally, for adults who choose to drink alcohol, drinking should not exceed moderate intake, and the calories from alcoholic beverages should be considered within overall calorie limits.[3]

Figure 2-8.
Typical Versus Nutrient-Dense Foods & Beverages

Achieving a healthy eating pattern means shifting typical food choices to more nutrient-dense options—that is, foods with important nutrients that aren't packed with extra calories or sodium. Nutrient-dense foods and beverages are naturally lean or low in solid fats and have little or no **added** solid fats, sugars, refined starches, or sodium.

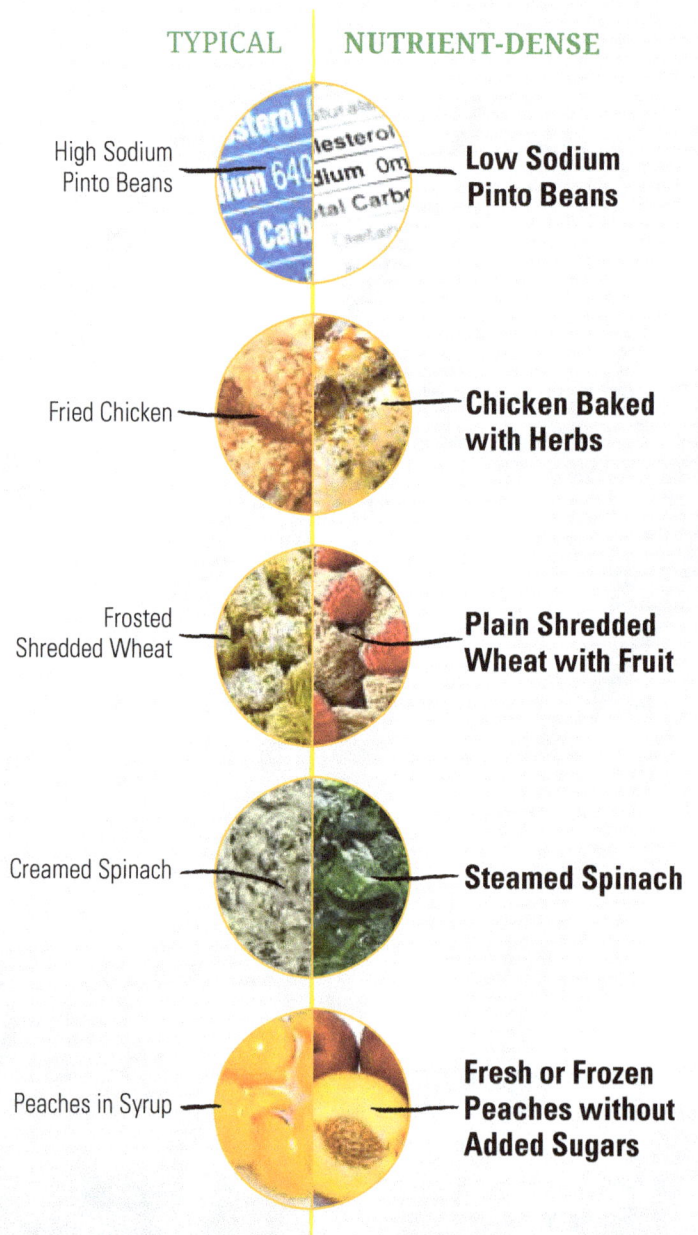

TYPICAL	NUTRIENT-DENSE
High Sodium Pinto Beans	**Low Sodium Pinto Beans**
Fried Chicken	**Chicken Baked with Herbs**
Frosted Shredded Wheat	**Plain Shredded Wheat with Fruit**
Creamed Spinach	**Steamed Spinach**
Peaches in Syrup	**Fresh or Frozen Peaches without Added Sugars**

[3] It is not recommended that individuals begin drinking or drink more for any reason. The amount of alcohol and calories in beverages varies and should be accounted for within the limits of healthy eating patterns. Alcohol should be consumed only by adults of legal drinking age. There are many circumstances in which individuals should not drink, such as during pregnancy. See Appendix 9. Alcohol for additional information.

Figure 2-9.

Average Intakes of Added Sugars as a Percent of Calories per Day by Age-Sex Group, in Comparison to the *Dietary Guidelines* Maximum Limit of Less than 10 Percent of Calories

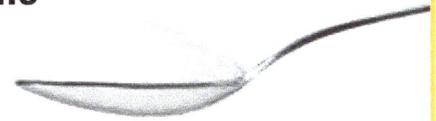

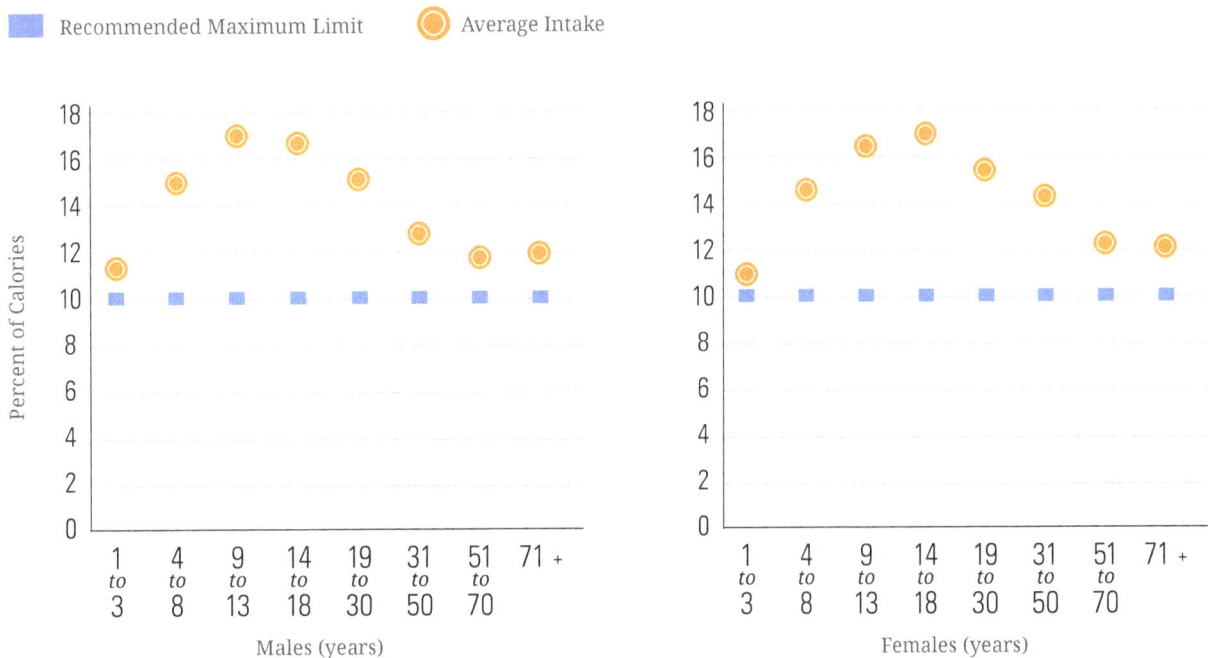

■ Recommended Maximum Limit   ● Average Intake

Males (years)

Percent of Calories							
1 to 3	4 to 8	9 to 13	14 to 18	19 to 30	31 to 50	51 to 70	71 +

Females (years)

Percent of Calories							
1 to 3	4 to 8	9 to 13	14 to 18	19 to 30	31 to 50	51 to 70	71 +

NOTE: The maximum amount of added sugars allowable in a Healthy U.S.-Style Eating Pattern at the 1,200-to-1,800 calorie levels is less than the *Dietary Guidelines* limit of 10 percent of calories. Patterns at these calorie levels are appropriate for many children and older women who are not physically active.

DATA SOURCE: What We Eat in America, NHANES 2007-2010 for average intakes by age-sex group.

The following sections describe total intakes compared to limits for these components, and the leading food categories contributing to this total.

Added Sugars

Current Intakes: Added sugars account on average for almost 270 calories, or more than 13 percent of calories per day in the U.S. population. As shown in **Figure 2-9**, intakes as a percent of calories are particularly high among children, adolescents, and young adults. The major source of added sugars in typical U.S. diets is beverages, which include soft drinks, fruit drinks, sweetened coffee and tea, energy drinks, alcoholic beverages, and flavored waters (**Figure 2-10**). Beverages account for almost half (47%) of all added sugars consumed by the U.S. population (**Figure 2-10**). The other major source of added sugars is snacks and sweets, which includes grain-based desserts such as cakes, pies, cookies, brownies, doughnuts, sweet rolls, and pastries; dairy desserts such as ice cream, other frozen desserts, and puddings; candies; sugars; jams; syrups; and sweet toppings. Together, these food categories make up more than 75 percent of intake of all added sugars.

Figure 2-10.
Food Category Sources of Added Sugars in the U.S. Population Ages 2 Years & Older

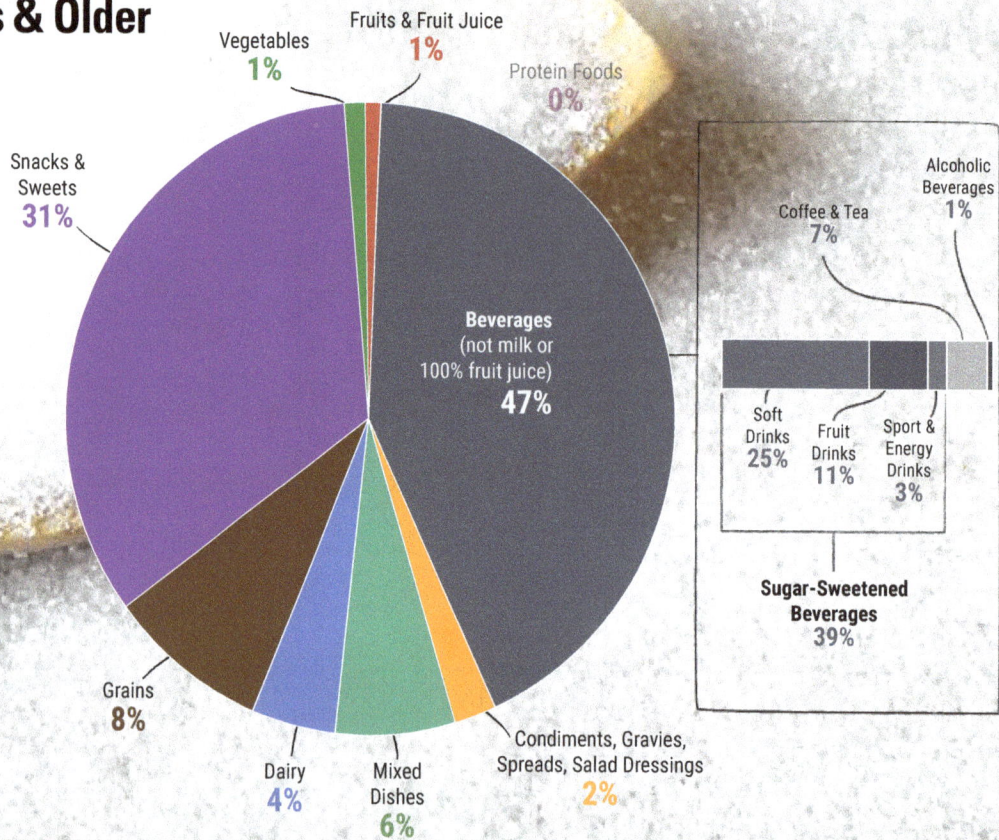

Vegetables
1%

Fruits & Fruit Juice
1%

Protein Foods
0%

Snacks & Sweets
31%

Beverages (not milk or 100% fruit juice)
47%

Grains
8%

Dairy
4%

Mixed Dishes
6%

Condiments, Gravies, Spreads, Salad Dressings
2%

Coffee & Tea
7%

Alcoholic Beverages
1%

Soft Drinks
25%

Fruit Drinks
11%

Sport & Energy Drinks
3%

Sugar-Sweetened Beverages
39%

DATA SOURCE: What We Eat in America (WWEIA) Food Category analyses for the 2015 Dietary Guidelines Advisory Committee. Estimates based on day 1 dietary recalls from WWEIA, NHANES 2009-2010.

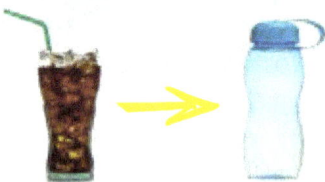

Shift To Reduce Added Sugars Consumption to Less Than 10 Percent of Calories per Day:[4]

Individuals have many potential options for reducing the intake of added sugars. Strategies include choosing beverages with no added sugars, such as water, in place of sugar-sweetened beverages, reducing portions of sugar-sweetened beverages, drinking these beverages less often, and selecting beverages low in added sugars. Low-fat or fat-free milk or 100% fruit or vegetable juice also can be consumed within recommended amounts in place of sugar-sweetened beverages. Additional strategies include limiting or decreasing portion size of grain-based and dairy desserts and sweet snacks and choosing unsweetened or no-sugar-added versions of canned fruit, fruit sauces (e.g., applesauce), and yogurt. The use of high-intensity sweeteners as a replacement for added sugars is discussed in Chapter 1 in the Added Sugars section.

Saturated Fats

Current Intakes: Current average intakes of saturated fats are 11 percent of calories. Only 29 percent of individuals in the United States

[4] See Added Sugars section of Chapter 1 for more information and Appendix 3. USDA Food Patterns: Healthy U.S.-Style Eating Patterns for specific limits on calories that remain after meeting food group recommendation in nutrient-dense forms ("calorie limits for other uses").

consume amounts of saturated fats consistent with the limit of less than 10 percent of calories (see **Figure 2-1**). As shown in **Figure 2-11**, average intakes do not vary widely across age-sex groups. Average intakes for both adult men and adult women are at 10.9 percent, and the average intake for children ranges from 11.1 percent up to 12.6 percent of calories.

The mixed dishes food category is the major source of saturated fats in the United States (**Figure 2-12**), with 35 percent of all saturated fats coming from mixed dishes, especially those dishes containing cheese, meat, or both. These include burgers, sandwiches, and tacos; pizza; rice, pasta, and grain dishes; and meat, poultry, and seafood dishes. The other food categories that provide the most saturated fats in current diets are snacks and sweets, protein foods, and dairy products.

Shift To Reduce Saturated Fats Intake to Less Than 10 Percent of Calories Per Day:

Individuals should aim to shift food choices from those high in saturated fats to those high in polyunsaturated and monounsaturated fats. Strategies to lower saturated fat intake include reading food labels to choose packaged foods lower in saturated fats and higher in polyunsaturated and monounsaturated fats, choosing lower fat forms of foods and beverages that contain solid fats (e.g., fat-free or low-fat milk instead of 2% or whole milk; low-fat cheese instead of regular cheese; lean rather than fatty cuts of meat), and consuming smaller portions of foods higher in saturated fats or consuming them less often. One realistic option is to change ingredients in mixed dishes to increase the amounts of vegetables, whole grains, lean meat, and low-fat or fat-free cheese, in place of some of the fatty meat and/or regular cheese in the dish. Additional strategies include preparing foods using oils that are high in polyunsaturated and monounsaturated fats, rather than solid fats, which are high in saturated fats (see Chapter 1, **Figure 1-2**), and using oil-based dressings and spreads on foods instead of those made from solid fats (e.g., butter, stick margarine, cream cheese) (see Solid Fats call-out box).

Figure 2-11.
Average Intakes of Saturated Fats as a Percent of Calories per Day by Age-Sex Groups, in Comparison to the *Dietary Guidelines* Maximum Limit of Less Than 10 Percent of Calories

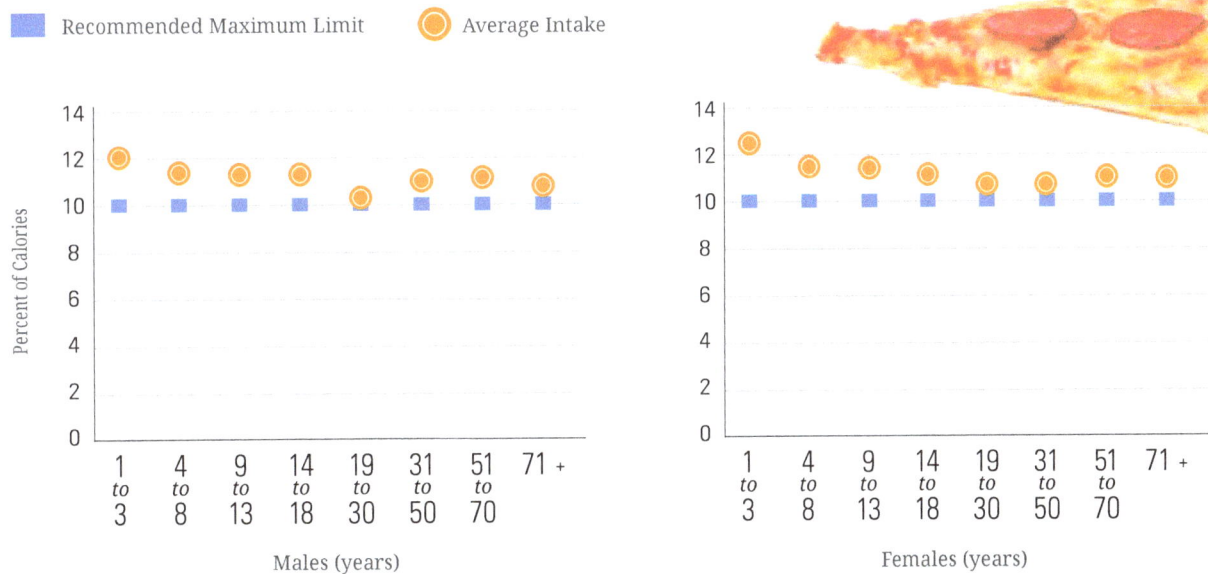

Legend: ■ Recommended Maximum Limit   ● Average Intake

Males (years): age groups 1 to 3, 4 to 8, 9 to 13, 14 to 18, 19 to 30, 31 to 50, 51 to 70, 71+

Females (years): age groups 1 to 3, 4 to 8, 9 to 13, 14 to 18, 19 to 30, 31 to 50, 51 to 70, 71+

DATA SOURCE: What We Eat in America, NHANES 2007-2010 for average intakes by age-sex group.

Figure 2-12.
Food Category Sources of Saturated Fats in the U.S. Population Ages 2 Years & Older

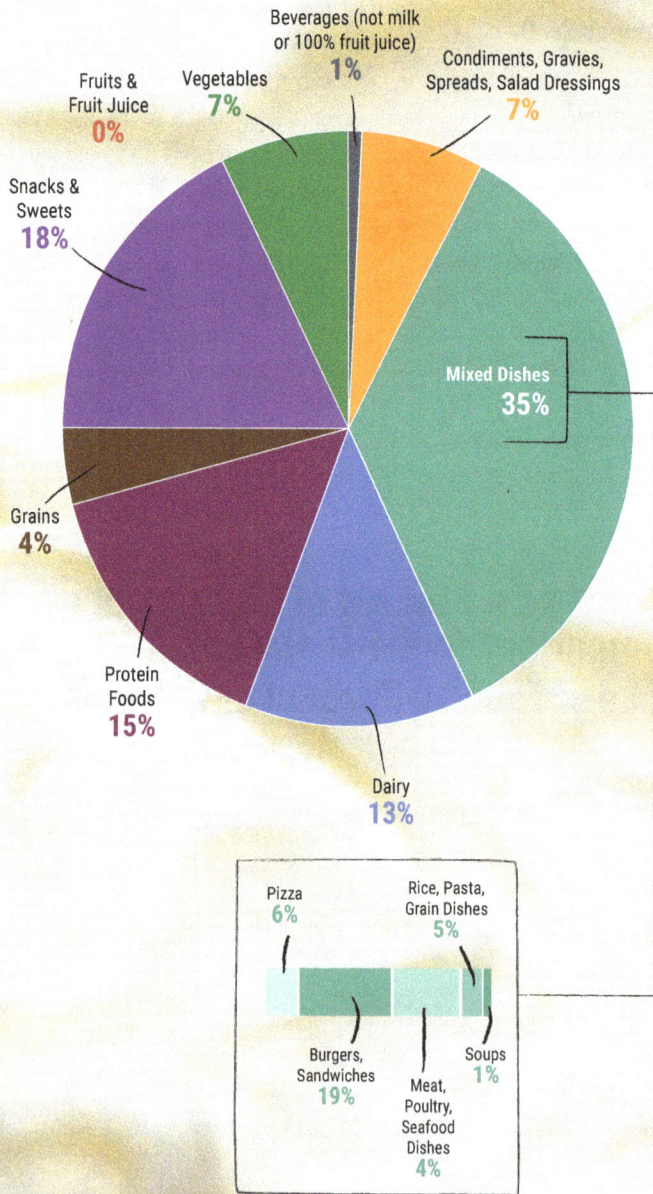

Beverages (not milk or 100% fruit juice) **1%**

Condiments, Gravies, Spreads, Salad Dressings **7%**

Vegetables **7%**

Fruits & Fruit Juice **0%**

Snacks & Sweets **18%**

Mixed Dishes **35%**

Grains **4%**

Protein Foods **15%**

Dairy **13%**

Pizza **6%**

Rice, Pasta, Grain Dishes **5%**

Burgers, Sandwiches **19%**

Meat, Poultry, Seafood Dishes **4%**

Soups **1%**

DATA SOURCE: What We Eat in America (WWEIA) Food Category analyses for the 2015 Dietary Guidelines Advisory Committee. Estimates based on day 1 dietary recalls from WWEIA, NHANES 2009-2010.

Solid Fats

Solid fats are the fats found in meats, poultry, dairy products, hydrogenated vegetable oils, and some tropical oils. They contain more saturated fatty acids and less mono- and polyunsaturated fatty acids, compared to oils (see Chapter 1, **Figure 1-2**). Solid fats, including the tropical oils, are solid at room temperature. In some foods, such as whole milk, the solid fat (butterfat) is suspended in the fluid milk by the process of homogenization.

The purpose of discussing solid fats in addition to saturated fats is that, apart from the effects of saturated fats on cardiovascular disease risk, solid fats are abundant in diets in the United States and contribute substantially to excess calorie intake. Solid fats, consumed as part of foods or added to foods, account for more than 325 calories or more than 16 percent of calories per day, on average, for the U.S. population but provide few nutrients. Food category sources of solid fats are similar to those for saturated fats: mixed dishes, snacks and sweets, protein foods, and dairy. Because solid fats are the major source of saturated fats, the strategies for reducing the intake of solid fats parallel the recommendations for reducing saturated fats. These strategies include choosing packaged foods lower in saturated fats; shifting from using solid fats to oils in preparing foods; choosing dressings and spreads that are made from oils rather than solid fats; reducing overall intake of solid fats by choosing lean or low-fat versions of meats, poultry, and dairy products; and consuming smaller portions of foods higher in solid fats or consuming them less often.

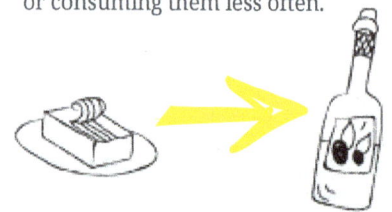

Figure 2-13.

Average Intake of Sodium in Milligrams per Day by Age-Sex Groups, Compared to Tolerable Upper Intake Levels (UL)

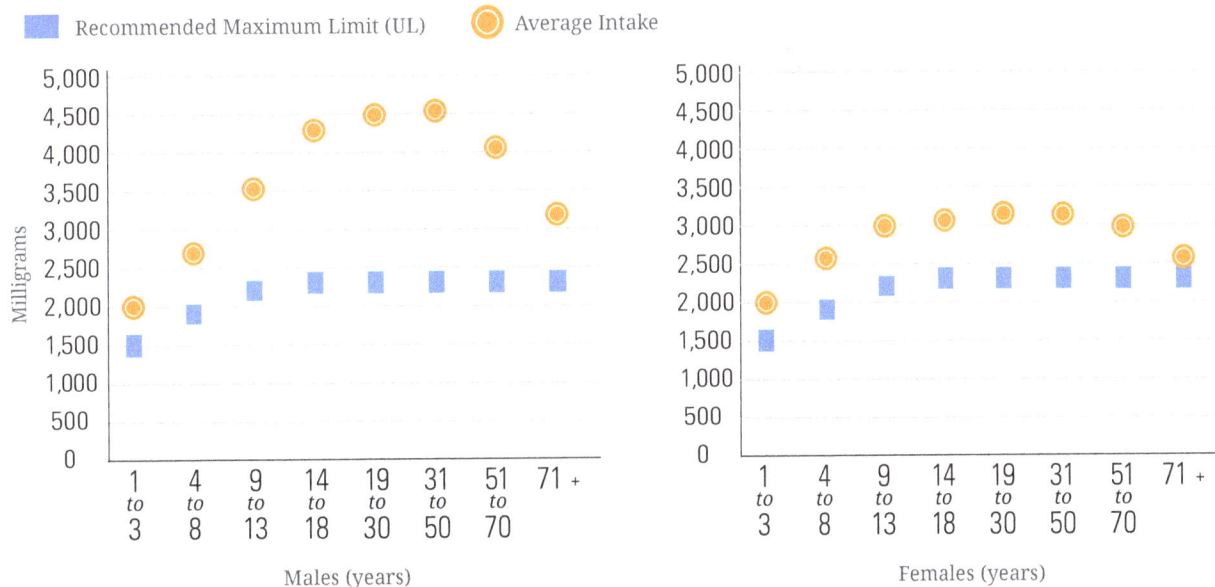

■ Recommended Maximum Limit (UL)   ◉ Average Intake

Males (years)

Females (years)

DATA SOURCES: What We Eat in America, NHANES 2007-2010 for average intakes by age-sex group. Institute of Medicine Dietary Reference Intakes for Tolerable Upper Intake Levels (UL).

Sodium

Current Intakes: As shown in **Figure 2-13**, average intakes of sodium are high across the U.S. population compared to the Tolerable Upper Intake Levels (ULs). Average intakes for those ages 1 year and older is 3,440 mg per day. Average intakes are generally higher for men than women. For all adult men, the average intake is 4,240 mg, and for adult women, the average is 2,980 mg per day. Only a small proportion of total sodium intake is from sodium inherent in foods or from salt added in home cooking or at the table. Most sodium consumed in the United States comes from salts added during commercial food processing and preparation.

Sodium is found in foods from almost all food categories (**Figure 2-14**). Mixed dishes—including burgers, sandwiches, and tacos; rice, pasta, and grain dishes; pizza; meat, poultry, and seafood dishes; and soups—account for almost half of the sodium consumed in the United States. The foods in many of these categories are often commercially processed or prepared.

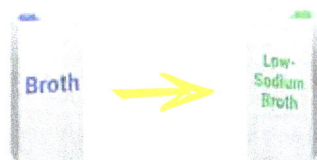

Shift Food Choices To Reduce Sodium Intake:[5]

Because sodium is found in so many foods, careful choices are needed in all food groups to reduce intake. Strategies to lower sodium intake include using the Nutrition Facts label to compare sodium content of foods and choosing the product with less sodium and buying low-sodium, reduced sodium, or no-salt-added versions of products when available. Choose fresh, frozen (no sauce or seasoning), or no-salt-added canned vegetables, and fresh poultry, seafood, pork, and lean meat, rather than processed meat and poultry. Additional strategies include eating at home more often; cooking foods from scratch to control the sodium content of dishes; limiting sauces, mixes, and "instant" products, including flavored rice, instant noodles, and ready-made pasta; and flavoring foods with herbs and spices instead of salt.

[5] The recommendation to limit intake of sodium to less than 2,300 mg per day is the UL for individuals ages 14 years and older set by the IOM. The recommendations for children younger than 14 years of age are the IOM age- and sex-appropriate ULs (see Appendix 7. Nutritional Goals for Age-Sex Groups, Based on Dietary Reference Intakes and Dietary Guidelines Recommendations).

Figure 2-14.

Food Category Sources of Sodium in the U.S. Population Ages 2 Years & Older

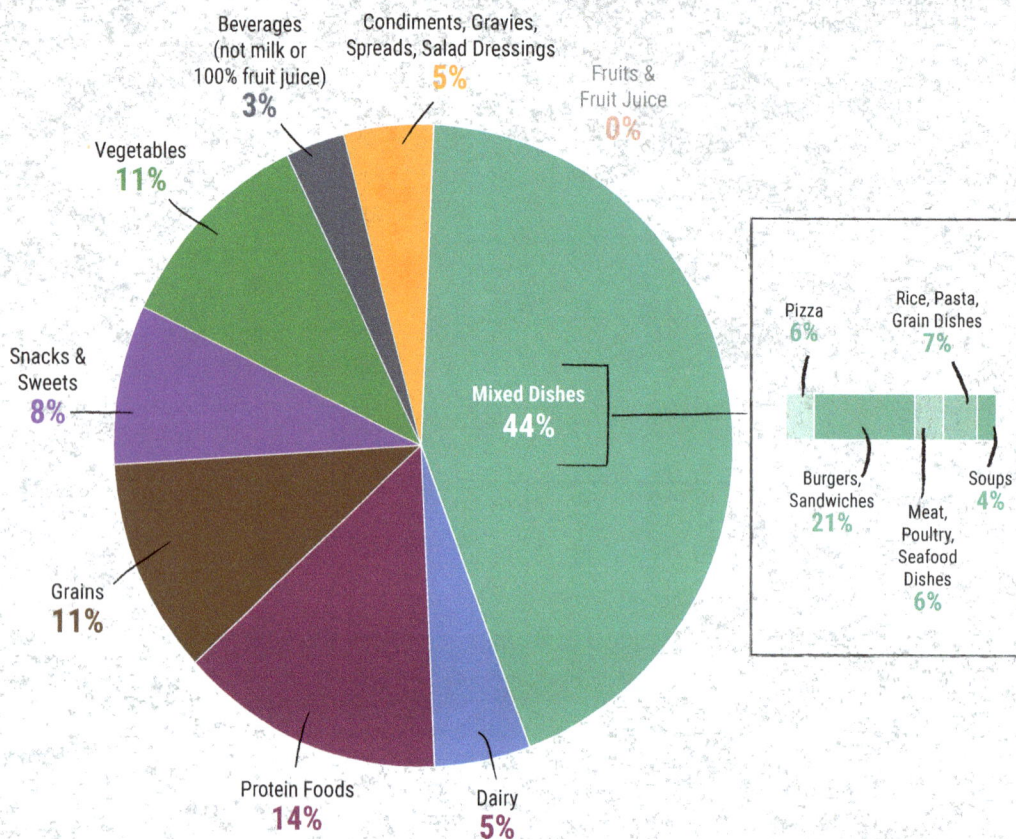

Beverages
(not milk or
100% fruit juice)
3%

Condiments, Gravies,
Spreads, Salad Dressings
5%

Fruits &
Fruit Juice
0%

Vegetables
11%

Snacks &
Sweets
8%

Grains
11%

Protein Foods
14%

Dairy
5%

Mixed Dishes
44%

Pizza
6%

Rice, Pasta,
Grain Dishes
7%

Burgers,
Sandwiches
21%

Meat,
Poultry,
Seafood
Dishes
6%

Soups
4%

DATA SOURCE: What We Eat in America (WWEIA) Food Category analyses for the 2015 Dietary Guidelines Advisory Committee. Estimates based on day 1 dietary recalls from WWEIA, NHANES 2009-2010.

Alcohol

In 2011, approximately 56 percent of U.S. adults 21 years of age and older were current drinkers, meaning that they had consumed alcohol in the past month; and 44 percent were not current drinkers. Current drinkers include 19 percent of all adults who consistently limited intake to moderate drinking, and 37 percent of all adults who did not. Drinking in greater amounts than moderation was more common among men, younger adults, and non-Hispanic whites. Two in three adult drinkers do not limit alcohol intake to moderate amounts one or more times per month.

The *Dietary Guidelines* does not recommend that individuals begin drinking or drink more for any reason. The amount of alcohol and calories in beverages varies and should be accounted for within the limits of healthy eating patterns. Alcohol should be consumed only by adults of legal drinking age. There are many circumstances in which individuals should not drink, such as during pregnancy. See Chapter 1 and Appendix 9. Alcohol for additional information.

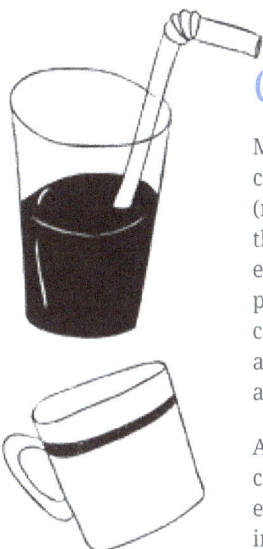

Caffeine

More than 95 percent of all adults consume caffeine from foods and/or beverages.[6] Average intakes of caffeine among adults, by age-sex group, range from 110 mg (females ages 19 to 30 years) up to 260 mg (males ages 51 to 70 years) per day. These amounts are substantially less than 400 mg per day, which is the upper amount associated with moderate coffee consumption that can be incorporated into healthy eating patterns. However, daily intakes of caffeine exceed 400 mg per day for a small percent of the adult population. The 90th percentile of caffeine intake for men ages 31 to 70 years, and the 95th percentile of caffeine intake for women ages 31 years and older, is greater than 400 mg per day. Caffeine sources for adults are largely from coffee and tea, which provide about 70 to 90 percent of total caffeine intake across all adult age groups.

Average intakes for children (5 to 32 mg/d) and adolescents (63 to 80 mg/d) are low. Caffeine sources for children and adolescents are distributed among coffee, tea, and sugar-sweetened beverages in roughly equal amounts. For young children, desserts and sweets also are a notable source of caffeine from certain ingredients such as chocolate, but intake of caffeine is low from all sources.

Underconsumed Nutrients & Nutrients of Public Health Concern

In addition to helping reduce chronic disease risk, the shifts in eating patterns described in this chapter can help individuals meet nutrient needs. This is especially important for nutrients that are currently underconsumed. Although the majority of Americans consume sufficient amounts of most nutrients, some nutrients are consumed by many individuals in amounts below the Estimated Average Requirement or Adequate Intake levels. These include potassium, dietary fiber, choline, magnesium, calcium, and vitamins A, D, E, and C. Iron also is underconsumed by adolescent girls and women ages 19 to 50 years. Low intakes for most of these nutrients occur within the context of unhealthy overall eating patterns, due to low intakes of the food groups—vegetables, fruits, whole grains, and dairy—that contain these nutrients. Shifts to increase the intake of these food groups can move intakes of these underconsumed nutrients closer to recommendations.

Of the underconsumed nutrients, calcium, potassium, dietary fiber, and vitamin D are considered nutrients of public health concern because low intakes are associated with health concerns. For young children, women capable of becoming pregnant, and women who are pregnant, low intake of iron also is of public health concern.

***Shift* to eating more vegetables, fruits, whole grains, and dairy to increase intake of nutrients of public health concern.**

Low intakes of dietary fiber are due to low intakes of vegetables, fruits, and whole grains. Low intakes of potassium are due to low intakes of vegetables, fruits, and dairy. Low intakes of calcium are due to low intakes of dairy. If a healthy eating pattern, such as the Healthy U.S.-Style Eating Pattern, is consumed, amounts of calcium and dietary fiber will meet recommendations. Amounts of potassium will increase but depending on food choices may not meet the Adequate Intake recommendation. To increase potassium, focus on food choices with the most potassium, listed in Appendix 10. Food Sources of Potassium, such as white potatoes, beet greens, white beans, plain yogurt, and sweet potato.

Although amounts of vitamin D in the USDA Food Patterns are less than recommendations, vitamin D is unique in that sunlight on the skin enables the body to make vitamin D. Recommendations for vitamin D assume minimum sun exposure. Strategies to achieve higher levels of intake of dietary vitamin D include consuming seafood with higher amounts of vitamin D, such as salmon, herring, mackerel, and tuna, and more foods fortified with vitamin D, especially fluid milk, soy beverage (soymilk), yogurt, orange juice, and breakfast cereals. In some cases, taking a vitamin D supplement may be appropriate, especially when sunshine exposure is limited due to climate or the use of sunscreen.

The best food sources of potassium, calcium, vitamin D, and dietary fiber are found in Appendix 10, Appendix 11, Appendix 12, and Appendix 13, respectively.

Substantial numbers of women who are capable of becoming pregnant, including adolescent girls, are at risk of iron-deficiency anemia due to low intakes of

---

[6] Caffeine is a substance that is generally recognized as safe (GRAS) in cola-type beverages by the Food and Drug Administration for use by adults and children. For more information, see: Code of Federal Regulation Title 21, subchapter B, Part 182, Subpart B. Caffeine. U.S. Government Printing Office. November 23, 2015. Available at: http://www.ecfr.gov/cgi-bin/retrieveECFR?gp=1&SID=f8c3068e9ec0062a3b4078cfa6361cf6&ty=HTML&h=L&mc=true&r=SECTION&n=se21.3.182_11180. Accessed October 22, 2015.

iron. To improve iron status, women and adolescent girls should consume foods containing heme iron, such as lean meats, poultry, and seafood, which is more readily absorbed by the body. Additional iron sources include legumes (beans and peas) and dark-green vegetables, as well as foods enriched or fortified with iron, such as many breads and ready-to-eat cereals. Absorption of iron from non-heme sources is enhanced by consuming them along with vitamin C-rich foods. Women who are pregnant are advised to take an iron supplement when recommended by an obstetrician or other health care provider.

Beverages

Beverages are not always remembered or considered when individuals think about overall food intake. However, they are an important component of eating patterns. In addition to water, the beverages that are most commonly consumed include sugar-sweetened beverages, milk and flavored milk, alcoholic beverages, fruit and vegetable juices, and coffee and tea. Beverages vary in their nutrient and calorie content. Some, like water, do not contain any calories. Some, like soft drinks, contain calories but little nutritional value. Finally, some, like milk and fruit and vegetable juices, contain important nutrients such as calcium, potassium, and vitamin D, in addition to calories.

Beverages make a substantial contribution to total water needs as well as to nutrient and calorie intakes in most typical eating patterns. In fact, they account for almost 20 percent of total calorie intake. Within beverages, the largest source of calories is sweetened beverages, accounting for 35 percent of calories from beverages. Other major sources of calories from beverages are milk and milk drinks, alcoholic beverages, fruit and vegetable juices, and coffee and tea.

When choosing beverages, both the calories and nutrients they may provide are important considerations. Beverages that are calorie-free—especially water—or that contribute beneficial nutrients, such as fat-free and low-fat milk and 100% juice, should be the primary beverages consumed. Milk and 100% fruit juice should be consumed within recommended food group amounts and calorie limits. Sugar-sweetened beverages, such as soft drinks, sports drinks, and fruit drinks that are less than 100% juice, can contribute excess calories while providing few or no key nutrients. If they are consumed, amounts should be within overall calorie limits and limits for calories from added sugars (see Chapter 1). The use of high-intensity sweeteners, such as those used in "diet" beverages, as a replacement for added sugars is discussed in Chapter 1 in the Added Sugars section.

For adults who choose to drink alcohol, limits of only moderate intake (see Appendix 9) and overall calorie limits apply.[8] Coffee, tea, and flavored waters also can be selected, but calories from cream, added sugars, and other additions should be accounted for within the eating pattern.

Opportunities for Shifts in Food Choices

To support a healthy body weight, meet nutrient needs, and lessen the risk of chronic disease, shifts are needed in

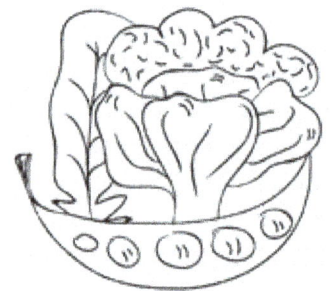

Folic Acid for Women Capable of Becoming Pregnant & Who Are Pregnant

The RDAs for folate are based on the prevention of folate deficiency, not on the prevention of neural tube defects. The RDA for adult women is 400 micrograms (mcg) Dietary Folate Equivalents (DFE)[7] and for women during pregnancy, 600 mcg DFE daily from all sources.

Folic acid fortification of enriched grain products in the United States has been successful in reducing the incidence of neural tube defects. Therefore, to prevent birth defects, all women capable of becoming pregnant are advised to consume 400 mcg of synthetic folic acid daily, from fortified foods and/or supplements. This recommendation is for an intake of synthetic folic acid in addition to the amounts of food folate contained in a healthy eating pattern. All enriched grains are fortified with synthetic folic acid. Sources of food folate include beans and peas, oranges and orange juice, and dark-green leafy vegetables, such as spinach and mustard greens.

[7] Dietary Folate Equivalents (DFE) adjust for the difference in bioavailability of food folate compared with synthetic folic acid. Food folate, measured as micrograms DFE, is less bioavailable than folic acid. 1 DFE = 1 mcg food folate = 0.6 mcg folic acid from supplements and fortified foods taken with meals.

[8] It is not recommended that individuals begin drinking or drink more for any reason. The amount of alcohol and calories in beverages varies and should be accounted for within the limits of healthy eating patterns. Alcohol should be consumed only by adults of legal drinking age. There are many circumstances in which individuals should not drink, such as during pregnancy. See Appendix 9 for additional information.

overall eating patterns—across and within food groups and from current typical choices to nutrient-dense options. Eating patterns are the result of choices on multiple eating occasions over time, both at home and away from home. As a result, individuals have many opportunities to make shifts to improve eating patterns.

The majority of the U.S. population consumes three meals a day plus more than one snack. Children ages 2 to 5 years are most likely to consume three meals a day, with 84 percent consuming three meals and most often, two or more snacks. In contrast, only half of adolescent females and young adult males consume three meals a day, but most also have two or more snacks per day. Also, among most age groups, 40 to 50 percent consume two to three snacks a day, and about one-third consume four or more snacks a day.

About two-thirds (67%) of the calories consumed by the U.S. population are purchased at a store, such as a grocery store or supermarket, and consumed in the home. However, Americans have increased the proportion of food they consume away from home from 18 percent in 1977-1978 to 33 percent in 2009-2010.

These data suggest that multiple opportunities to improve food choices exist throughout the day and in varied settings where food is obtained and consumed. Small shifts made at each of these many eating occasions over time can add up to real improvements in eating patterns.

Summary

The U.S. population, across almost every age and sex group, consumes eating patterns that are low in vegetables, fruits, whole grains, dairy, seafood, and oil and high in refined grains, added sugars, saturated fats, sodium, and for some age-sex groups, high in the meats, poultry, and eggs subgroup. Although most Americans urgently need to shift intakes to achieve the healthy eating patterns described in Chapter 1, young children and older Americans generally are closer to the recommendations than are adolescents and young adults. For some aspects of eating patterns, maintaining the intake levels of young children as they grow into adolescence and adulthood could result in healthy eating patterns across the lifespan and improved health over time.

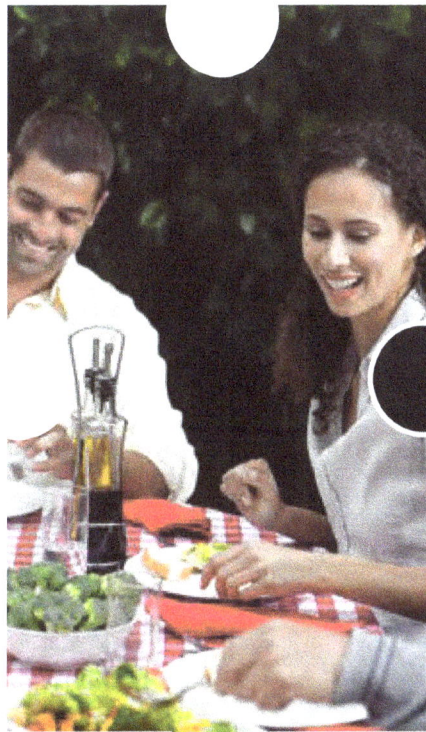

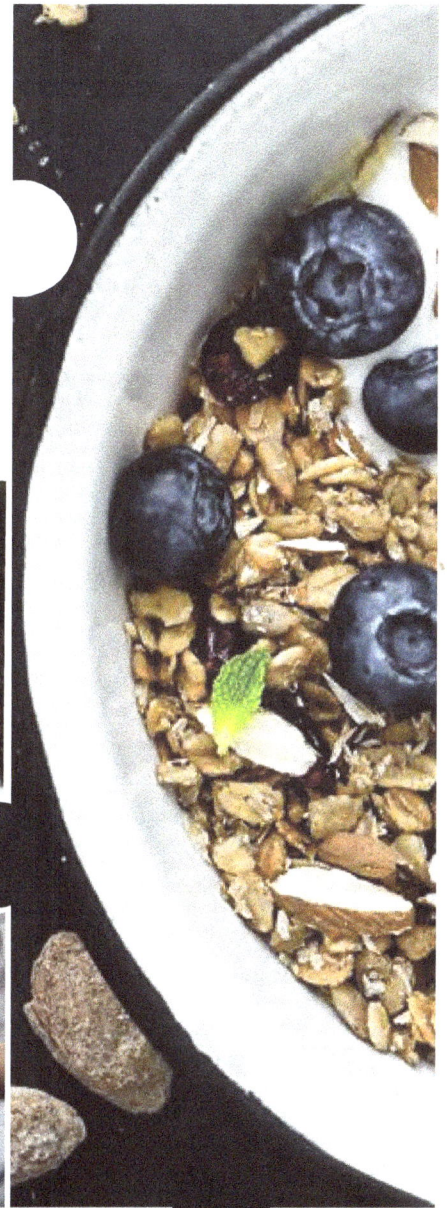

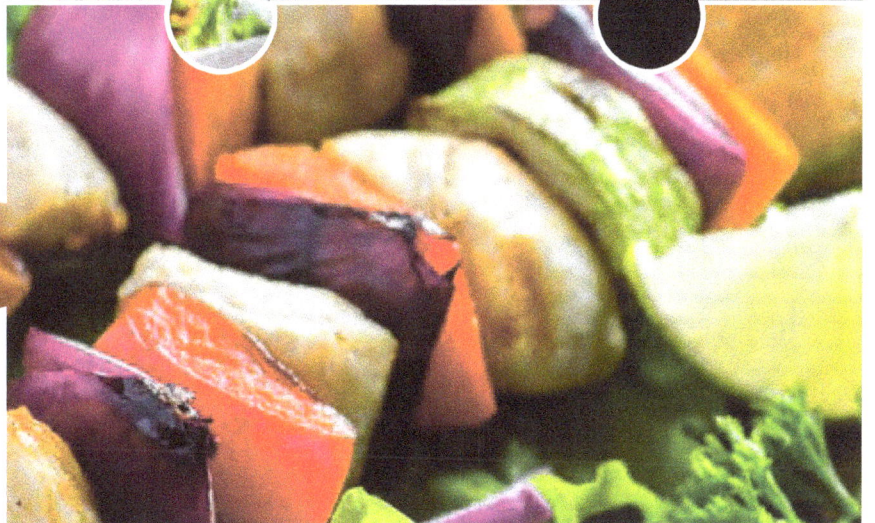

CHAPTER 3

Everyone Has a Role in Supporting Healthy Eating Patterns

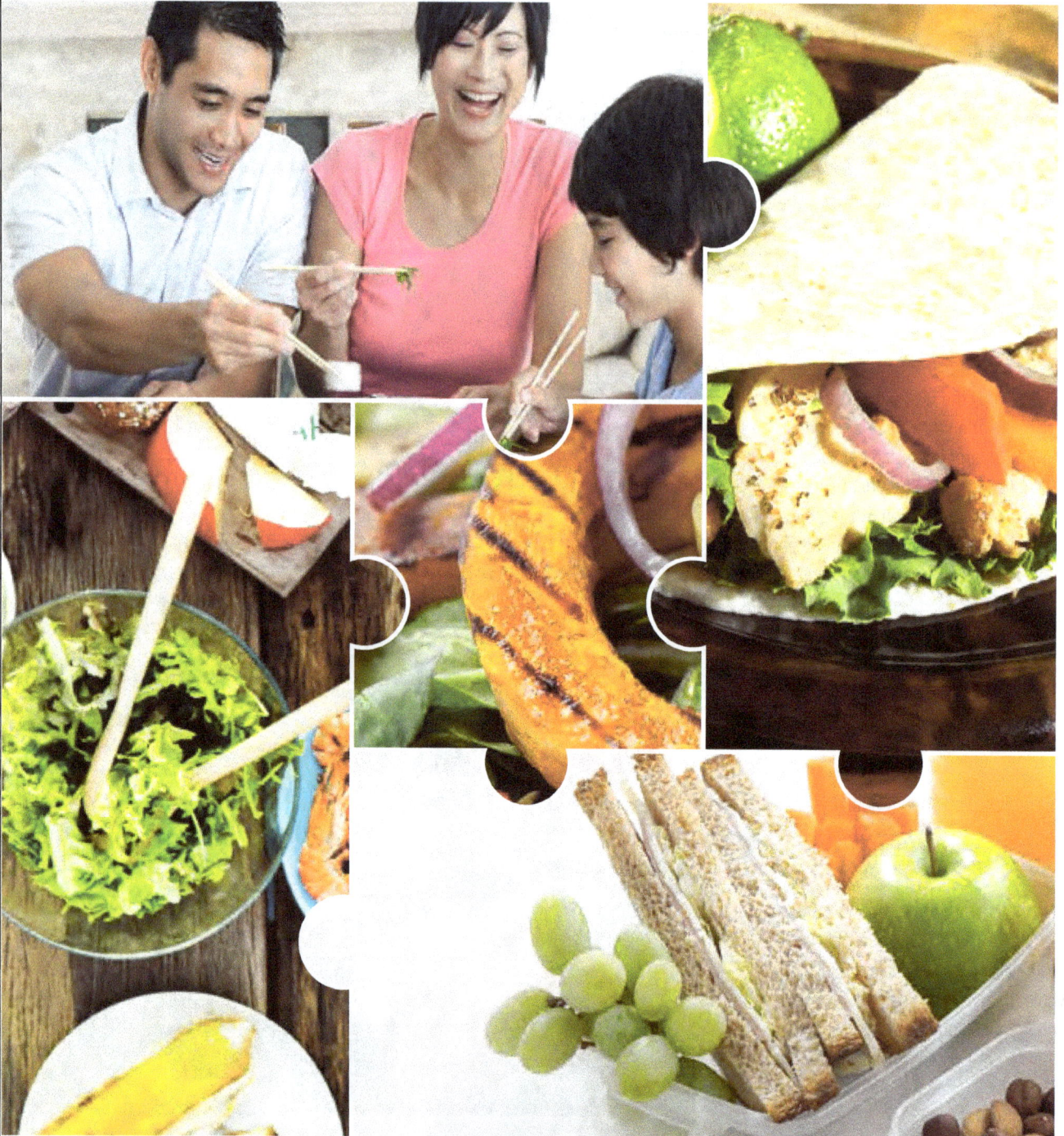

Introduction

The previous chapters describe the characteristics of healthy eating and physical activity patterns, and it is clear that across all population groups, the vast majority of people in the United States are not meeting these recommendations. In general, Americans are consuming too many calories, are not meeting food group and nutrient recommendations, and are not getting adequate physical activity. In practice, aligning with the *Dietary Guidelines* (see Aligning With the *Dietary Guidelines for Americans*: What Does This Mean in Practice? in the Introduction) at the population level requires broad, multisectoral coordination and collaboration. This collective action is needed to create a new paradigm in which healthy lifestyle choices at home, school, work, and in the community are easy, accessible, affordable, and normative. Everyone has a role in helping individuals shift their everyday food,[1] beverage, and physical activity choices to align with the *Dietary Guidelines*.

The *Dietary Guidelines* provides recommendations that professionals, especially policymakers, can translate into action to support individuals. This chapter discusses a number of considerations related to translating the *Dietary Guidelines* into action, including the significance of using multiple strategies across all segments of society to promote healthy eating and physical activity behaviors; the development of educational resources that deliver information in a way that is compelling, inspiring, empowering, and actionable for individuals; and the need to focus on individuals where they are making food and beverage choices.

About This Chapter

This chapter focuses on the fifth Guideline:

1. **Follow a healthy eating pattern across the lifespan.** All food and beverage choices matter. Choose a healthy eating pattern at an appropriate calorie level to help achieve and maintain a healthy body weight, support nutrient adequacy, and reduce the risk of chronic disease.

2. **Focus on variety, nutrient density, and amount.** To meet nutrient needs within calorie limits, choose a variety of nutrient-dense foods across and within all food groups in recommended amounts.

3. **Limit calories from added sugars and saturated fats and reduce sodium intake.** Consume an eating pattern low in added sugars, saturated fats, and sodium. Cut back on foods and beverages higher in these components to amounts that fit within healthy eating patterns.

4. **Shift to healthier food and beverage choices.** Choose nutrient-dense foods and beverages across and within all food groups in place of less healthy choices. Consider cultural and personal preferences to make these shifts easier to accomplish and maintain.

5. **Support healthy eating patterns for all.** Everyone has a role in helping to create and support healthy eating patterns in multiple settings nationwide, from home to school to work to communities.

The Social-Ecological Model (**Figure 3-1**) is used as a framework to illustrate how sectors, settings, social and cultural norms, and individual factors converge to influence food and physical activity choices. The chapter describes contextual factors that influence eating as well as physical activity behaviors and identifies opportunities for professionals, including policymakers, to implement strategies that can help individuals align with the *Dietary Guidelines*.

Creating & Supporting Healthy Choices

As shown in the Social-Ecological Model, a multitude of choices, messages, individual resources, and other factors affect the food and physical activity choices an individual makes, and these decisions are rarely made in isolation. The following section describes the various components in the Social-Ecological Model and how they play a role in influencing the decisions individuals make about foods and physical activity. Ideas for engaging these components in collaborative ways to influence individual decisions, and ultimately social and cultural norms and values to align with the *Dietary Guidelines*, are provided.

The Social-Ecological Model

Consistent evidence shows that implementing multiple changes at various levels of the Social-Ecological Model is effective in improving eating and physical activity behaviors. For example, strong evidence from studies with varying designs and generally consistent findings demonstrates that school policies designed to enhance the school food setting leads to improvements in the purchasing behavior of children, resulting in higher dietary quality of the food consumed during the school day. For adults, moderate evidence indicates

[1] If not specified explicitly, references to "foods" refer to "foods and beverages."

that worksite nutrition policies can improve dietary intake, and approaches targeting dietary intake and physical activity can favorably affect weight-related outcomes. These examples demonstrate how support and active engagement from various segments of society are needed to help individuals change their eating and physical activity behaviors and achieve positive outcomes. Approaches like these have the potential to improve population health if they can be incorporated into existing organizational structures and maintained over time. Among the components of the Social-Ecological Model, sectors and settings influence change at the population level and are addressed first in this discussion.

Sectors

Sectors include systems (e.g., governments, education, health care, and transportation), organizations (e.g., public health, community, and advocacy), and businesses and industries (e.g., planning and development, agriculture, food and beverage, retail, entertainment, marketing, and media).

Figure 3-1.
A Social-Ecological Model for Food & Physical Activity Decisions

The Social-Ecological Model can help health professionals understand how layers of influence intersect to shape a person's food and physical activity choices. The model below shows how various factors influence food and beverage intake, physical activity patterns, and ultimately health outcomes.

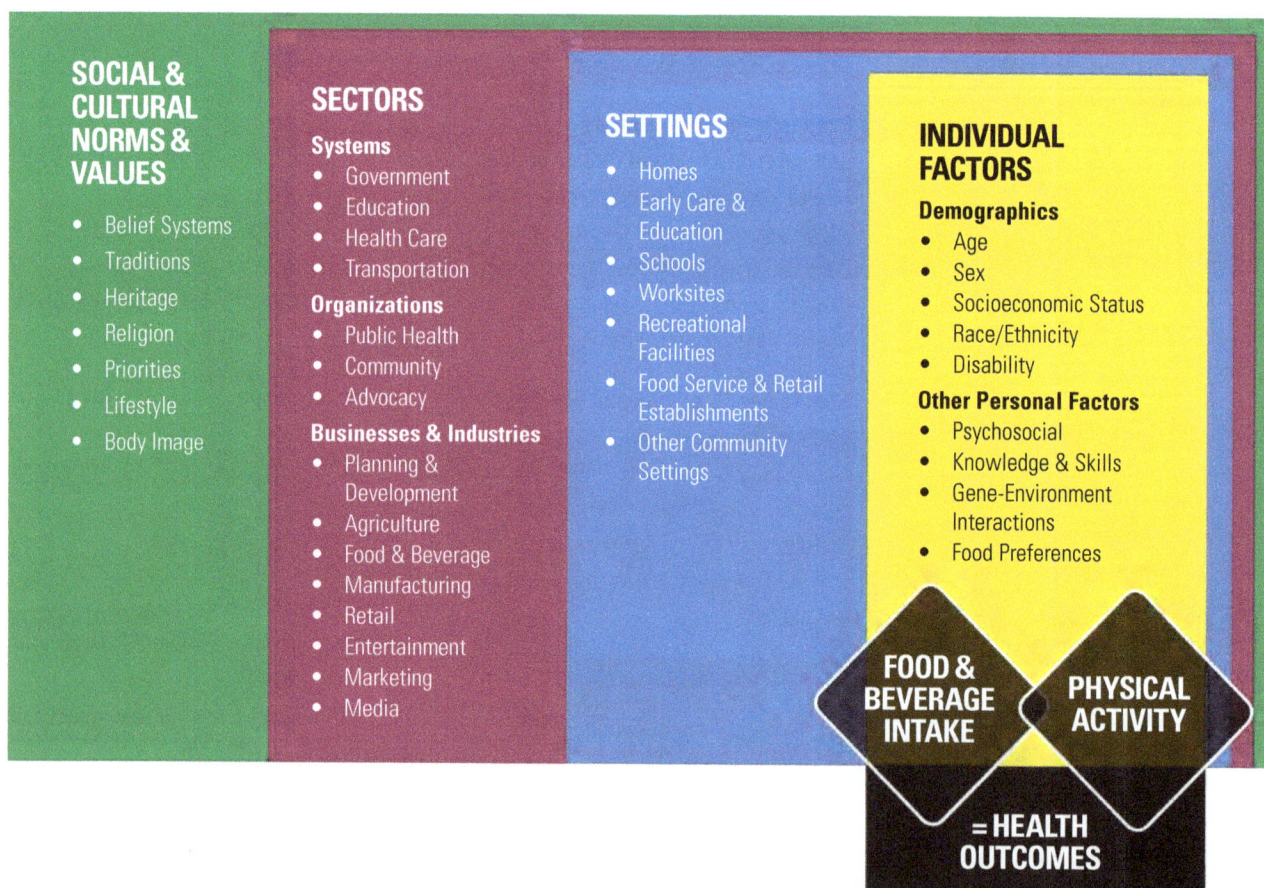

SOCIAL & CULTURAL NORMS & VALUES
- Belief Systems
- Traditions
- Heritage
- Religion
- Priorities
- Lifestyle
- Body Image

SECTORS

Systems
- Government
- Education
- Health Care
- Transportation

Organizations
- Public Health
- Community
- Advocacy

Businesses & Industries
- Planning & Development
- Agriculture
- Food & Beverage
- Manufacturing
- Retail
- Entertainment
- Marketing
- Media

SETTINGS
- Homes
- Early Care & Education
- Schools
- Worksites
- Recreational Facilities
- Food Service & Retail Establishments
- Other Community Settings

INDIVIDUAL FACTORS

Demographics
- Age
- Sex
- Socioeconomic Status
- Race/Ethnicity
- Disability

Other Personal Factors
- Psychosocial
- Knowledge & Skills
- Gene-Environment Interactions
- Food Preferences

FOOD & BEVERAGE INTAKE + **PHYSICAL ACTIVITY** = **HEALTH OUTCOMES**

DATA SOURCES: Adapted from: (1) Centers for Disease Control and Prevention. Division of Nutrition, Physical Activity, and Obesity. National Center for Chronic Disease Prevention and Health Promotion. Addressing Obesity Disparities: Social Ecological Model. Available at: http://www.cdc.gov/obesity/health_equity/addressingtheissue.html. Accessed October 19, 2015. (2) Institute of Medicine. Preventing Childhood Obesity: Health in the Balance, Washington (DC): The National Academies Press; 2005, page 85. (3) Story M, Kaphingst KM, Robinson O Brien R, Glanz K. Creating healthy food and eating environments: Policy and environmental approaches. Annu Rev Public Health 2008; 29:253-272.

These sectors all have an important role in helping individuals make healthy choices because they either influence the degree to which people have access to healthy food and/or opportunities to be physically active, or they influence social norms and values. Positive influences on social norms and values can occur through effective health promotion and marketing strategies.

Professionals in these sectors have many opportunities to identify and develop strategies that help individuals align their choices with the *Dietary Guidelines*. Strategies could include supporting policy and/or program changes, fostering coalitions and networks, developing or modifying products and menus, and/or creating opportunities to be physically active. To ensure widespread adoption of these sectoral efforts, complementary efforts can include training, education, and/or motivational strategies.

Settings

Individuals make choices in a variety of settings, both at home and away from home. Away-from-home settings include early care and education programs (e.g., child care, preschool), schools, worksites, community centers, and food retail and food service establishments. These organizational settings determine what foods are offered and what opportunities for physical activity are provided. Strategies to align with the *Dietary Guidelines* that are implemented in these settings can influence individual choices and have the potential for broader population-level impact if they are integrated with strategies by multiple sectors. In combination, sectors and settings can influence social norms and values.

Social & Cultural Norms & Values

Social and cultural *norms* are rules that govern thoughts, beliefs, and behaviors. They are shared assumptions of appropriate behaviors, based on the values of a society, and are reflected in everything from laws to personal expectations. With regard to nutrition and physical activity, examples of norms include preferences for certain types of foods, attitudes about acceptable ranges of body weight, and values placed on physical activity and health. Because norms and values are prevalent within a community or setting, changing them can be difficult. However, changes to sectors and settings—as previously discussed—can have a powerful effect on social and cultural norms and values over time and can align with the *Dietary Guidelines*.

Individual Factors

Individual factors are those that are unique to the individual, such as age, sex, socioeconomic status, race/ethnicity, the presence of a disability, as well as other influences, such as physical health, knowledge and skills, and personal preferences. Education to improve individual food and physical activity choices can be delivered by a wide variety of nutrition and physical activity professionals working alone or in multidisciplinary teams. Resources based on systematic reviews of scientific evidence, such as the *Dietary Guidelines* and the *Physical Activity Guidelines for Americans*, provide the foundation for nutrition and public health professionals to develop programs and materials that can help individuals enhance their knowledge, attitudes, and motivation to make healthy choices.

All food and beverage choices are part of an individual's eating pattern. Professionals can work with individuals in a variety of settings to adapt their choices to develop a healthy eating pattern tailored to accommodate physical health, cultural, ethnic, traditional, and personal preferences, as well as personal food budgets and other issues of accessibility. Eating patterns tailored to the individual are more likely to be motivating, accepted, and maintained over time, thereby having the potential to lead to meaningful shifts in dietary intake, and consequently, improved health.

Opportunities To Align Food Products & Menus With the *Dietary Guidelines*

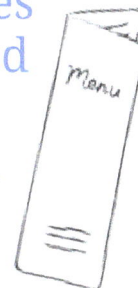

During the past few decades, food products and menus have notably evolved in response to consumer demands and public health concerns. The food and beverage and food service sectors and settings have a unique opportunity to continue to evolve and better align with the *Dietary Guidelines*. Reformulation and menu and retail modification opportunities that align with the *Dietary Guidelines* include offering more vegetables, fruits, whole grains, low-fat and fat-free dairy, and a greater variety of protein foods that are nutrient dense, while also reducing sodium and added sugars, reducing saturated fats and replacing them with unsaturated fats, and reducing added refined starches. Portion sizes also can be adapted to help individuals make choices that align with the *Dietary Guidelines*. Food manufacturers are encouraged to consider the entire composition of the food, and not just individual nutrients or ingredients when developing or reformulating products. Similarly, when developing or modifying menus or retail settings, establishments can consider the range of offerings both within and across food groups and other dietary components to determine whether the healthy options offered reflect the proportions in healthy eating patterns. In taking these actions, care should be taken to assess any potential unintended consequences so that as changes are made to better align with the *Dietary Guidelines*, undesirable changes are not introduced.

Meeting People Where They Are: Contextual Factors & Healthy Eating Patterns

As previously described, the Social-Ecological Model provides a framework for how individuals make food and physical activity choices (where, what, when, why, and how much) each day. Understanding individual choices and motivators and the context that affects them can help professionals identify which strategies are most likely to be effective to promote healthy choices aligned with the *Dietary Guidelines*.

The scientific literature has described a number of specific circumstances that can limit an individual's or family's capacity to choose a healthy diet. These contextual factors—food access, household food insecurity, and acculturation—are particularly important for millions of individuals living in the United States. As appropriate, professionals can consider these critical factors when developing strategies and providing education to enhance interventions.

Food Access

Having access to healthy, safe,[2] and affordable food choices is crucial for an individual to achieve a healthy eating pattern. Food access is influenced by diverse factors, including proximity to food retail outlets (e.g., distance to a store or the number of stores in an area), individual resources (e.g., income or personal transportation), and neighborhood-level resources (e.g., average income of the neighborhood and availability of public transportation). Race/ethnicity, socioeconomic status, geographic location, and the presence of a disability also may affect an individual's ability to access foods to support healthy eating patterns.

Innovative approaches are emerging to improve food access within communities. These include creating financing programs to incentivize grocery store development; increasing the availability of foods to support healthy eating patterns in retail outlets, including corner stores, bodegas, farmers markets, mobile markets, shelters, food banks, and community gardens/cooperatives; and creating new pathways for wholesale distribution through food hubs.

Food access is important in all settings where people make choices. Improving food access in settings, such as schools, worksites, early care and education programs, and food retail, may include changing organizational policies to improve the availability and provision of healthy food choices, developing or updating nutrition standards for food service operations, and educating customers about how to identify healthy choices, such as through point-of-purchase information. Changes to food options within a setting should not be done in isolation but with consideration of the overall mix of foods provided (e.g., in cafeterias, at meetings, in vending machines, concession stands and elsewhere).

To help everyone make choices that align with the *Dietary Guidelines*, professionals are encouraged to identify ways to improve food access. Ultimately, individual choices will be enhanced when sectors and settings ensure the accessibility of safe, affordable, and healthy food choices.

Household Food Insecurity

In the United States, about 48 million individuals live in households that experience food insecurity, which occurs when access to nutritionally adequate and safe food is limited or uncertain. Food insecurity can be temporary or persist over time. Living with food insecurity challenges a household's ability to obtain food and make healthy choices and can exacerbate stress and chronic disease risk. Government and nongovernment nutrition assistance programs play an essential role in providing food and educational resources to help participants make healthy food choices within their budget. Food insecurity persists in the United States, and maintaining current programs, networks, and partnerships is crucial in addressing the problem. Exploring innovative new strategies could provide opportunities to reach more individuals, families, and households experiencing food insecurity. For example, sectors can create networks and partnerships to deliver food and other resources to reach people who are in need and when community services are scarce. Individuals who are supported in this way are better able to obtain and make healthy food choices that align with the *Dietary Guidelines*.

Acculturation

The United States continues to evolve as a nation of individuals and families who emigrate from other countries. Individuals who come to this country may adopt the attitudes, values, customs, beliefs, and behaviors of a new culture as well as its dietary habits. Healthy eating patterns are designed to be flexible in order to accommodate traditional and cultural foods. Individuals are encouraged to retain the healthy aspects of their eating and physical activity patterns and avoid adopting behaviors that are less healthy. Professionals can help individuals or population groups by recognizing cultural diversity and developing programs and materials that are responsive and appropriate to their belief systems, lifestyles and practices, traditions, and other needs.

[2] See Appendix 14. Food Safety Principles and Guidance for guidance on food safety principles and practices.

Multi-Component Versus Multi-Level Strategies To Influence Food & Physical Activity Choices

Evidence demonstrates that both multi-component and multi-level changes must be implemented to effectively influence public health. Multi-component changes are those that use a *combination of strategies* to promote behavior change. These strategies can be employed across or within different settings. For example, a multi-component obesity prevention program at an early care and education center could target classroom education around nutrition and physical activity, ensure the continued nutritional quality of meals and snacks served, make improvements to the mealtime setting, increase opportunities for active play, and initiate active outreach to parents about making positive changes at home.

Multi-level changes are those that *target change at the individual level as well as additional levels*, such as in community, school, and retail settings. For example, strategies to reduce sodium intake could include providing individual education on how to interpret sodium information on food labels or restaurant menus (e.g., sodium versus salt), reformulating foods and meals to reduce sodium content in retail and food service establishments, and conducting public health campaigns to promote the importance of reducing sodium intake.

Many strategies for implementing these types of multi-component and multi-level actions have shown promise to positively influence food and physical activity choices. For example, moderate evidence indicates that multi-component school-based programs can improve dietary intake and weight status of school-aged children. Fundamental to the success of such actions is tailoring programs to meet the needs of the individual, the community, and/or the organization so as to increase the chances of affecting social and cultural norms and values over time.

Strategies for Action

To shift from current eating patterns to those that align with the *Dietary Guidelines*, collective action across all segments of society is needed. As previously described, these actions must involve a broad range of sectors, occur across a variety of settings, and address the needs of individuals, families, and communities. These actions include identifying and addressing successful approaches for change; improving knowledge of what constitutes healthy eating and physical activity patterns; enhancing access to adequate amounts of healthy, safe, and affordable food choices; and promoting change in social and cultural norms and values to embrace, support, and maintain healthy eating and physical activity behaviors.

The following examples of strategies exemplify the concerted action needed. It is important to note that no one strategy is likely to be the primary driver to improve individual and population lifestyle choices. Evidence demonstrates that multiple changes both within and across all levels of the Social-Ecological Model are needed to increase the effectiveness of interventions.

Sectors—Examples Include:

- Foster partnerships with food producers, suppliers, and retailers to increase access to foods that align with the *Dietary Guidelines*.

- Promote the development and availability of food products that align with the *Dietary Guidelines* in food retail and food service establishments.

- Identify and support policies and/or programs that promote healthy eating and physical activity patterns.

- Encourage participation in physical activity programs offered in various settings.

Settings—Examples Include:

- Expand access to healthy, safe, and affordable food choices that align with the *Dietary Guidelines* and provide opportunities for engaging in physical activity.

- Adopt organizational changes and practices, including those that increase the availability, accessibility, and consumption of foods that align with the *Dietary Guidelines*.

- Provide nutrition assistance programs that support education and promotional activities tailored to the needs of the community.

- Implement educational programs tailored to individuals and change organization practices, approaches, and/or policies to support healthy food choices where food decisions are being made, including at early care and education programs, schools, worksites, and other community settings.

- Encourage opportunities in the workplace for regular physical activity through active commuting, activity breaks, and walking meetings.

Using MyPlate as a Guide To Support Healthy Eating Patterns

The *Dietary Guidelines* is developed and written for a professional audience. Therefore, its translation into actionable consumer messages and resources is crucial to help individuals, families, and communities achieve healthy eating patterns. MyPlate is one such example (**Figure 3-2**). MyPlate is used by professionals across multiple sectors to help individuals become more aware of and educated about making healthy food and beverage choices over time. Created to be used in various settings and to be adaptable to the needs of specific population groups, the MyPlate symbol and its supporting consumer resources at ChooseMyPlate.gov bring together the key elements of healthy eating patterns, translating the *Dietary Guidelines* into key consumer messages that are used in educational materials and tools for the public.

Figure 3-2.
Implementation of the *Dietary Guidelines* Through MyPlate

MyPlate, MyWins.

Find your healthy eating style and maintain it for a lifetime. This means:

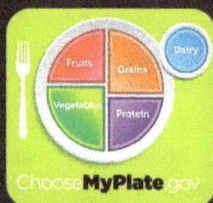

Everything you eat and drink over time matters.

The right mix can help you be healthier in the future.

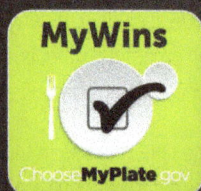

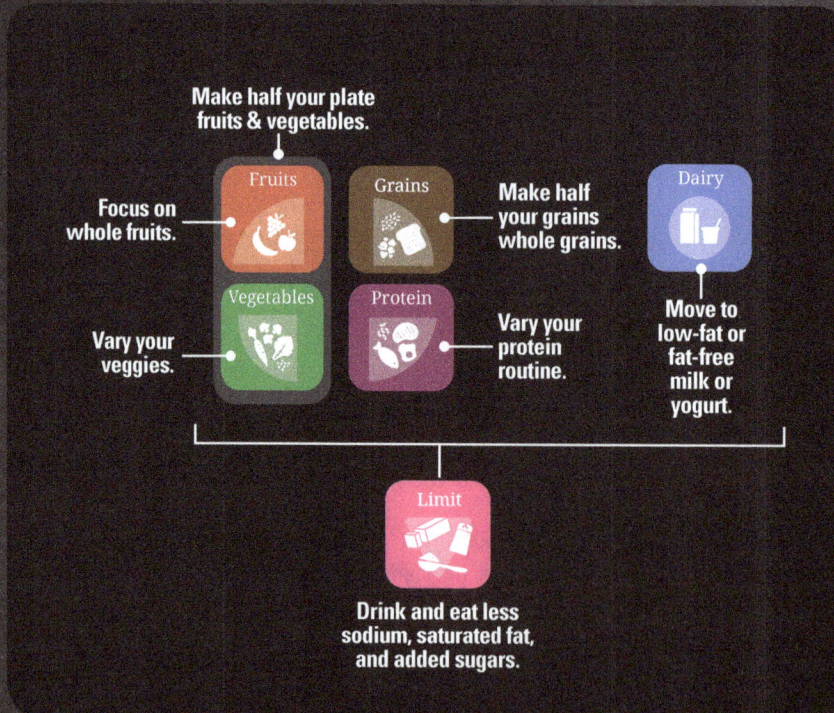

Make half your plate fruits & vegetables.

Focus on whole fruits.

Vary your veggies.

Make half your grains whole grains.

Vary your protein routine.

Move to low-fat or fat-free milk or yogurt.

Limit — Drink and eat less sodium, saturated fat, and added sugars.

MyWins
ChooseMyPlate.gov

Start with small changes to make healthier choices you can enjoy.
Visit Choose**MyPlate**.gov for more tips, tools, and information.

Figure 3-3.
Strategies To Align Settings With the *2015-2020 Dietary Guidelines*

Americans make food and beverage choices in a variety of settings at home, at work, and at play. Aligning these settings with the *2015-2020 Dietary Guidelines* will not only influence individual choices—it can also have broader population level impact when multiple sectors commit to make changes together.

HOME

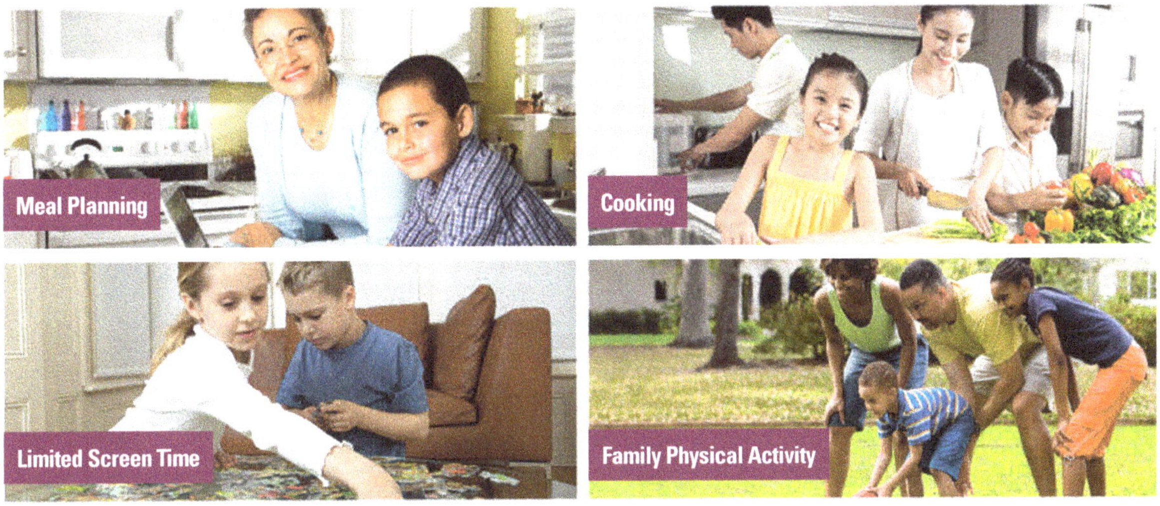

Meal Planning

Cooking

Limited Screen Time

Family Physical Activity

SCHOOL

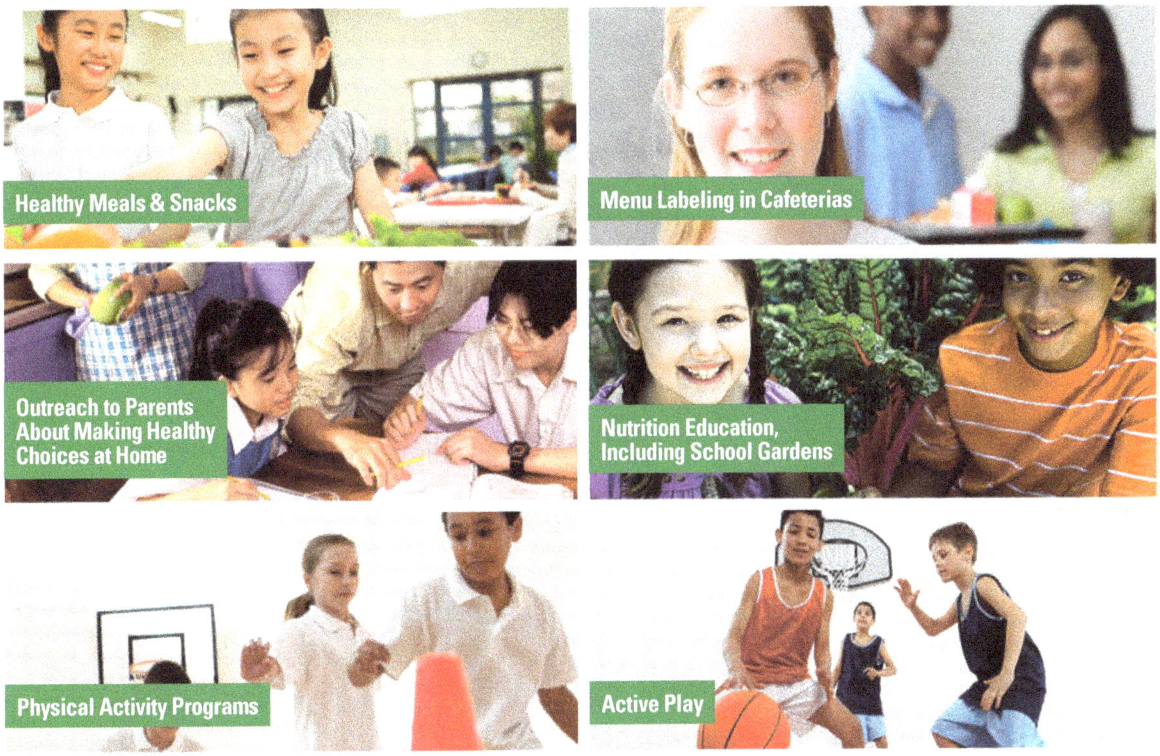

Healthy Meals & Snacks

Menu Labeling in Cafeterias

Outreach to Parents About Making Healthy Choices at Home

Nutrition Education, Including School Gardens

Physical Activity Programs

Active Play

Figure 3-3. *(continued...)*

Strategies To Align Settings With the *2015-2020 Dietary Guidelines*

Americans make food and beverage choices in a variety of settings at home, at work, and at play. Aligning these settings with the *2015-2020 Dietary Guidelines* will not only influence individual choices—it can also have broader population level impact when multiple sectors commit to make changes together.

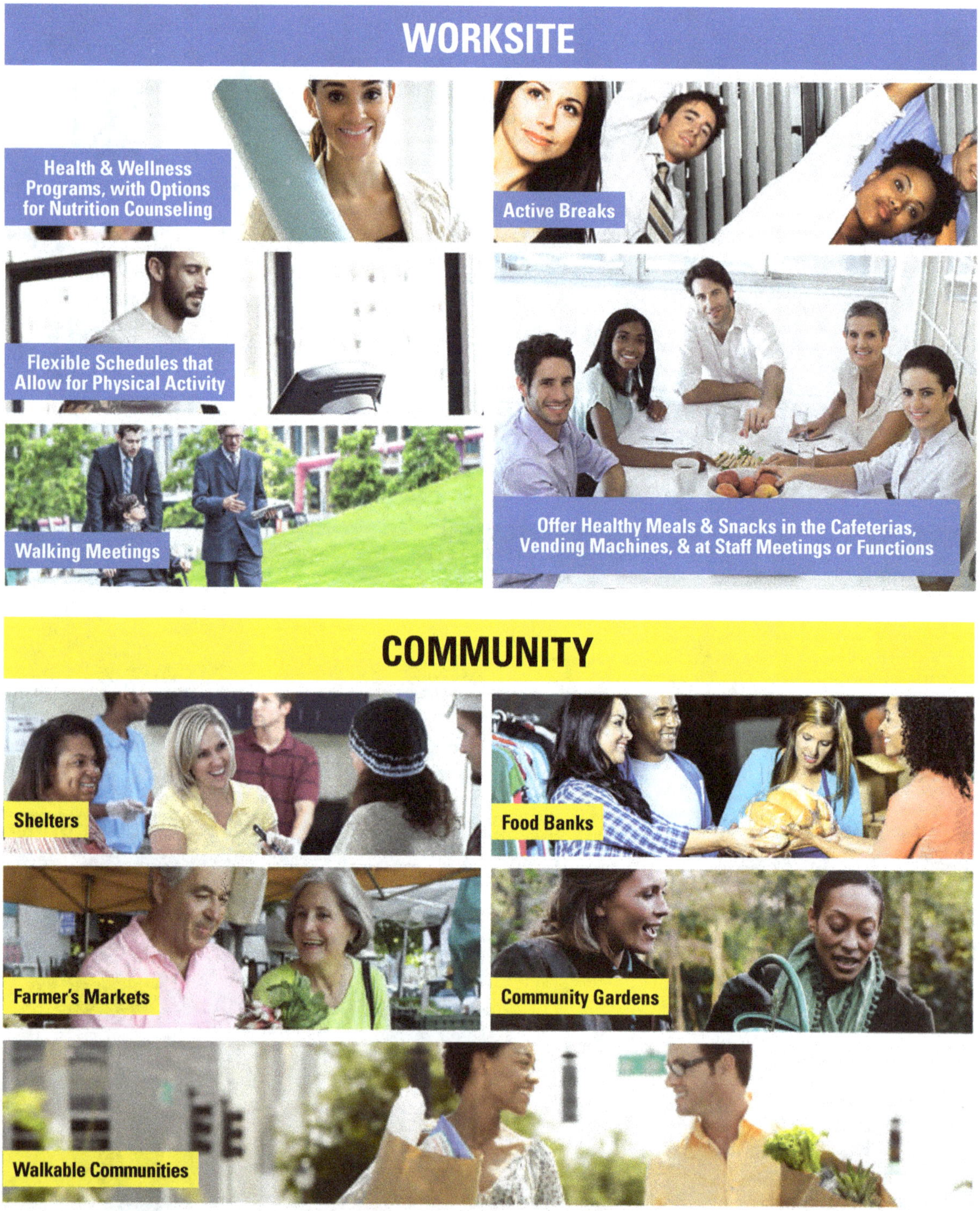

WORKSITE

Health & Wellness Programs, with Options for Nutrition Counseling

Active Breaks

Flexible Schedules that Allow for Physical Activity

Walking Meetings

Offer Healthy Meals & Snacks in the Cafeterias, Vending Machines, & at Staff Meetings or Functions

COMMUNITY

Shelters

Food Banks

Farmer's Markets

Community Gardens

Walkable Communities

FOOD RETAIL

Outreach to Consumers About Making Healthy Changes

Access to Healthy Food Options

Access to Healthy Food Choices

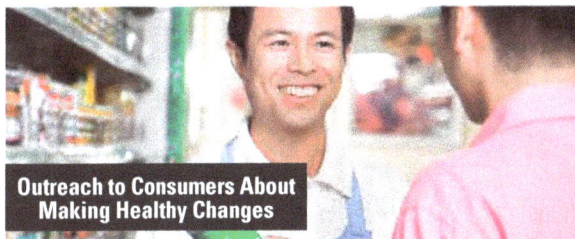

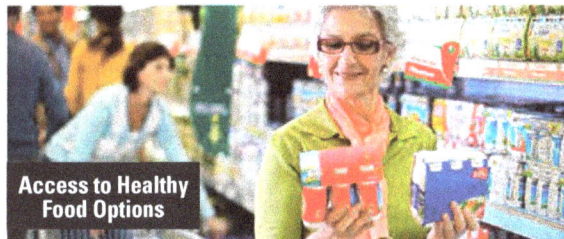

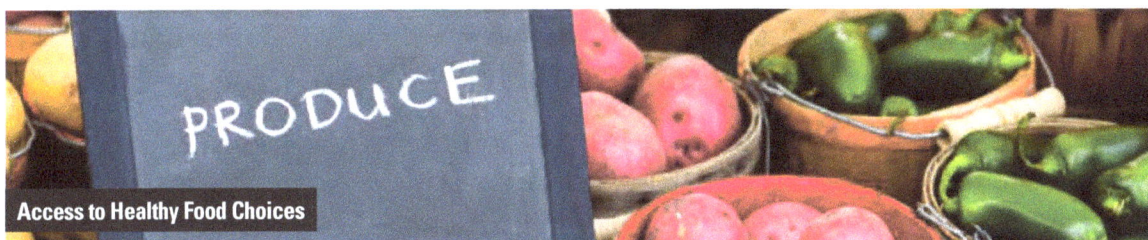

Professionals Working With Individuals—Examples Include:

- Help individuals become more aware of the foods and beverages that make up their own or their family's eating patterns and identify areas, such as modifying recipes and/or food selections, where they can make shifts to align with the *Dietary Guidelines*.

- Teach skills like gardening, cooking, meal planning, and label reading that help support healthy eating patterns.

- Suggest ways that individuals can model healthy eating behaviors for friends and family members.

- Develop plans to help individuals limit screen time and time spent being sedentary and increase physical activity to meet the *Physical Activity Guidelines for Americans*.

This is not an all-inclusive list; many strategies are available that can result in shifts to improve dietary intake and, ultimately, improve health. Professionals should help individuals understand that they can adapt their choices to create healthy eating patterns that encompass all foods and beverages, meet food group and nutrient needs, and stay within calorie limits.

Summary

Concerted efforts among professionals within communities, businesses and industries, organizations, governments, and other segments of society are needed to support individuals and families in making lifestyle choices that align with the *Dietary Guidelines*. Professionals have an important role in leading disease-prevention efforts within their organizations and communities to make healthy eating and regular physical activity an organizational and societal norm. Changes at multiple levels of the Social-Ecological Model are needed, and these changes, in combination and over time, can have a meaningful impact on the health of current and future generations.

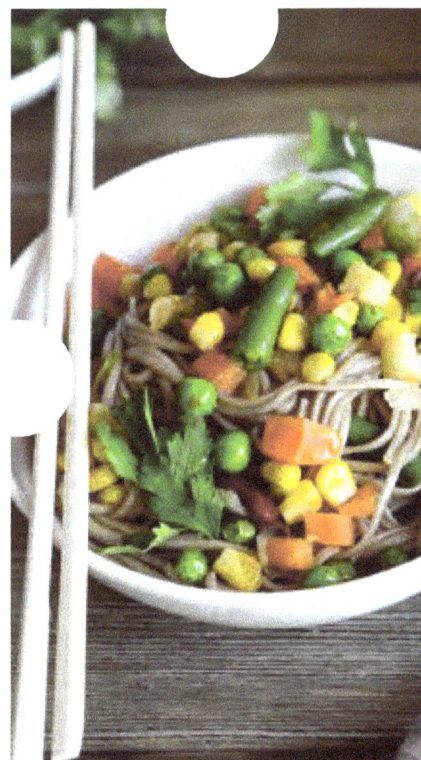

Appendix 1.

Physical Activity Guidelines for Americans

In addition to consuming a healthy eating pattern, regular physical activity is one of the most important things Americans can do to improve their health. The *Physical Activity Guidelines for Americans*,[1] released by the U.S. Department of Health and Human Services, provides a comprehensive set of recommendations for Americans on the amounts and types of physical activity needed each day. Adults need at least 150 minutes of moderate-intensity physical activity and should perform muscle-strengthening exercises on 2 or more days each week. Youth ages 6 to 17 years need at least 60 minutes of physical activity per day, including aerobic, muscle-strengthening, and bone-strengthening activities (see **Table A1-1** for additional details). Just as individuals can achieve a healthy eating pattern in a variety of ways that meet their personal and cultural preferences, they can engage in regular physical activity in a variety of ways throughout the day and by choosing activities they enjoy. **Table A1-2** provides a list of Federal resources, including handouts, online assessments, trackers, and interactive websites. These can be used to help motivate consumer audiences to make healthy physical activity choices.

Table A1-1.
Physical Activity Guidelines for Americans Recommendations

Age	Recommendations
6 to 17 Years	Children and adolescents should do 60 minutes (1 hour) or more of physical activity daily. • **Aerobic:** Most of the 60 or more minutes a day should be either moderate[a]- or vigorous-intensity[b] aerobic physical activity, and should include vigorous-intensity physical activity at least 3 days a week. • **Muscle-strengthening:**[c] As part of their 60 or more minutes of daily physical activity, children and adolescents should include muscle-strengthening physical activity on at least 3 days of the week. • **Bone-strengthening:**[d] As part of their 60 or more minutes of daily physical activity, children and adolescents should include bone-strengthening physical activity on at least 3 days of the week. • It is important to encourage young people to participate in physical activities that are appropriate for their age, that are enjoyable, and that offer variety.

[1] U.S. Department of Health and Human Services. *2008 Physical Activity Guidelines for Americans.* Washington (DC): U.S. Department of Health and Human Services; 2008. ODPHP Publication No. U0036. Available at: http://www.health.gov/paguidelines. Accessed August 6, 2015.

Age	Recommendations
18 to 64 Years	• All adults should avoid inactivity. Some physical activity is better than none, and adults who participate in any amount of physical activity gain some health benefits. • For substantial health benefits, adults should do at least 150 minutes (2 hours and 30 minutes) a week of moderate-intensity, or 75 minutes (1 hour and 15 minutes) a week of vigorous-intensity aerobic physical activity, or an equivalent combination of moderate- and vigorous-intensity aerobic activity. Aerobic activity should be performed in episodes of at least 10 minutes, and preferably, it should be spread throughout the week. • For additional and more extensive health benefits, adults should increase their aerobic physical activity to 300 minutes (5 hours) a week of moderate-intensity, or 150 minutes a week of vigorous-intensity aerobic physical activity, or an equivalent combination of moderate- and vigorous-intensity activity. Additional health benefits are gained by engaging in physical activity beyond this amount. • Adults should also include muscle-strengthening activities that involve all major muscle groups on 2 or more days a week.
65 Years & Older	• Older adults should follow the adult guidelines. When older adults cannot meet the adult guidelines, they should be as physically active as their abilities and conditions will allow. • Older adults should do exercises that maintain or improve balance if they are at risk of falling. • Older adults should determine their level of effort for physical activity relative to their level of fitness. • Older adults with chronic conditions should understand whether and how their conditions affect their ability to do regular physical activity safely.

[a] Moderate-intensity physical activity: Aerobic activity that increases a person's heart rate and breathing to some extent. On a scale relative to a person's capacity, moderate-intensity activity is usually a 5 or 6 on a 0 to 10 scale. Brisk walking, dancing, swimming, or bicycling on a level terrain are examples.

[b] Vigorous-intensity physical activity: Aerobic activity that greatly increases a person's heart rate and breathing. On a scale relative to a person's capacity, vigorous-intensity activity is usually a 7 or 8 on a 0 to 10 scale. Jogging, singles tennis, swimming continuous laps, or bicycling uphill are examples.

[c] Muscle-strengthening activity: Physical activity, including exercise that increases skeletal muscle strength, power, endurance, and mass. It includes strength training, resistance training, and muscular strength and endurance exercises.

[d] Bone-strengthening activity: Physical activity that produces an impact or tension force on bones, which promotes bone growth and strength. Running, jumping rope, and lifting weights are examples.

SOURCE: Adapted from U.S. Department of Health and Human Services. *2008 Physical Activity Guidelines for Americans.* Washington (DC): U.S. Department of Health and Human Services; 2008. Available at: http://www.health.gov/paguidelines. Accessed August 6, 2015.

Table A1-2.
Federal Physical Activity Resources

Program/Initiative	Lead Office	Website
Physical Activity Guidelines for Americans	Office of Disease Prevention and Health Promotion (ODPHP)	www.health.gov/paguidelines
Healthfinder.gov (Consumer Resources)	ODPHP	www.healthfinder.gov
Healthy People 2020 (Physical Activity National Objectives)	ODPHP	www.healthypeople.gov
Let's Move!	Office of the First Lady	www.letsmove.gov
Step it Up! The Surgeon General's Call to Action to Promote Walking and Walkable Communities	Office of the Surgeon General	www.surgeongeneral.gov
I Can Do It, You Can Do It	President's Council on Fitness, Sports & Nutrition (PCFSN)	www.fitness.gov
Presidential Youth Fitness Program	PCFSN	www.pyfp.org/index.shtml
The President's Challenge	PCFSN	www.presidentschallenge.org
The President's Challenge Adult Fitness Test	PCFSN	www.adultfitnesstest.org
Physical Activity Guidelines for Americans Youth Toolkit	U.S. Centers for Disease Control and Prevention (CDC)	www.cdc.gov/healthyschools/physicalactivity/guidelines.htm
BAM! Body and Mind (Focused on Tweens)	CDC	www.cdc.gov/bam

Program/Initiative	Lead Office	Website
We Can! (Ways to Enhance Childhood Nutrition and Physical Activity)	National Institutes of Health (NIH) National Heart, Lung, and Blood Institute	www.nhlbi.nih.gov/health/educational/wecan
Go4Life (Focused on Older Adults)	NIH National Institute on Aging	https://go4life.nia.nih.gov/
SuperTracker	U.S. Department of Agriculture	www.supertracker.usda.gov
National Physical Activity Plan (NPAP)*	NPAP Alliance	www.physicalactivityplan.org

* The National Physical Activity Plan is not a product of the Federal Government. However, a number of Federal officers were involved in the development of the Plan.

Appendix 2.

Estimated Calorie Needs per Day, by Age, Sex, & Physical Activity Level

The total number of calories a person needs each day varies depending on a number of factors, including the person's age, sex, height, weight, and level of physical activity. In addition, a need to lose, maintain, or gain weight and other factors affect how many calories should be consumed. Estimated amounts of calories needed to maintain calorie balance for various age and sex groups at three different levels of physical activity are provided in **Table A2-1**. These estimates are based on the Estimated Energy Requirements (EER) equations, using reference heights (average) and reference weights (healthy) for each age-sex group. For children and adolescents, reference height and weight vary. For adults, the reference man is 5 feet 10 inches tall and weighs 154 pounds. The reference woman is 5 feet 4 inches tall and weighs 126 pounds.

Estimates range from 1,600 to 2,400 calories per day for adult women and 2,000 to 3,000 calories per day for adult men. Within each age and sex category, the low end of the range is for sedentary individuals; the high end of the range is for active individuals. Due to reductions in basal metabolic rate that occur with aging, calorie needs generally decrease for adults as they age. Estimated needs for young children range from 1,000 to 2,000 calories per day, and the range for older children and adolescents varies substantially from 1,400 to 3,200 calories per day, with boys generally having higher calorie needs than girls. These are only estimates, and approximations of individual calorie needs can be aided with online tools such as those available at www.supertracker.usda.gov.

Table A2-1.

Estimated Calorie Needs per Day, by Age, Sex, & Physical Activity Level

Males

Age	Sedentary[a]	Moderately Active[b]	Active[c]
2	1,000	1,000	1,000
3	1,000	1,400	1,400
4	1,200	1,400	1,600
5	1,200	1,400	1,600
6	1,400	1,600	1,800
7	1,400	1,600	1,800
8	1,400	1,600	2,000

Females[d]

Age	Sedentary[a]	Moderately Active[b]	Active[c]
2	1,000	1,000	1,000
3	1,000	1,200	1,400
4	1,200	1,400	1,400
5	1,200	1,400	1,600
6	1,200	1,400	1,600
7	1,200	1,600	1,800
8	1,400	1,600	1,800

Males

Age	Sedentary[a]	Moderately Active[b]	Active[c]
9	1,600	1,800	2,000
10	1,600	1,800	2,200
11	1,800	2,000	2,200
12	1,800	2,200	2,400
13	2,000	2,200	2,600
14	2,000	2,400	2,800
15	2,200	2,600	3,000
16	2,400	2,800	3,200
17	2,400	2,800	3,200
18	2,400	2,800	3,200
19-20	2,600	2,800	3,000
21-25	2,400	2,800	3,000
26-30	2,400	2,600	3,000
31-35	2,400	2,600	3,000
36-40	2,400	2,600	2,800
41-45	2,200	2,600	2,800
46-50	2,200	2,400	2,800
51-55	2,200	2,400	2,800
56-60	2,200	2,400	2,600
61-65	2,000	2,400	2,600
66-70	2,000	2,200	2,600
71-75	2,000	2,200	2,600
76 & Up	2,000	2,200	2,400

Females[d]

Age	Sedentary[a]	Moderately Active[b]	Active[c]
9	1,400	1,600	1,800
10	1,400	1,800	2,000
11	1,600	1,800	2,000
12	1,600	2,000	2,200
13	1,600	2,000	2,200
14	1,800	2,000	2,400
15	1,800	2,000	2,400
16	1,800	2,000	2,400
17	1,800	2,000	2,400
18	1,800	2,000	2,400
19-20	2,000	2,200	2,400
21-25	2,000	2,200	2,400
26-30	1,800	2,000	2,400
31-35	1,800	2,000	2,200
36-40	1,800	2,000	2,200
41-45	1,800	2,000	2,200
46-50	1,800	2,000	2,200
51-55	1,600	1,800	2,200
56-60	1,600	1,800	2,200
61-65	1,600	1,800	2,000
66-70	1,600	1,800	2,000
71-75	1,600	1,800	2,000
76 & Up	1,600	1,800	2,000

[a] Sedentary means a lifestyle that includes only the physical activity of independent living.

[b] Moderately Active means a lifestyle that includes physical activity equivalent to walking about 1.5 to 3 miles per day at 3 to 4 miles per hour, in addition to the activities of independent living.

[c] Active means a lifestyle that includes physical activity equivalent to walking more than 3 miles per day at 3 to 4 miles per hour, in addition to the activities of independent living.

[d] Estimates for females do not include women who are pregnant or breastfeeding.

SOURCE: Institute of Medicine. Dietary Reference Intakes for Energy, Carbohydrate, Fiber, Fat, Fatty Acids, Cholesterol, Protein, and Amino Acids. Washington (DC): The National Academies Press; 2002.

Appendix 3.

USDA Food Patterns: Healthy U.S.-Style Eating Pattern

The Healthy U.S.-Style Pattern is based on the types and proportions of foods Americans typically consume, but in nutrient-dense forms and appropriate amounts. It is designed to meet nutrient needs while not exceeding calorie requirements and while staying within limits for overconsumed dietary components.

The methodology used to develop and update this Pattern continues to be grounded in that of the food guides USDA has developed for the last 30 years. This methodology includes using current food consumption data to determine the mix and proportions of foods to include in each group, using current food composition data to select a nutrient-dense representative for each food, and calculating nutrient profiles for each food group using these nutrient-dense representative foods. As would be expected, most foods in their nutrient-dense forms do contain some sodium and saturated fatty acids. In a few cases, such as whole-wheat bread, the most appropriate representative in current Federal databases contains a small amount of added sugars. Detailed information about the representative foods, nutrient profiles, and Patterns is available on the USDA Center for Nutrition Policy and Promotion website.[1]

Amounts of each food group and subgroup are adjusted as needed, within the limits of the range of typical consumption when possible, to meet nutrient and *Dietary Guidelines* standards while staying within the limits for calories and overconsumed dietary components. Standards for nutrient adequacy aim to meet the Recommended Dietary Allowances (RDA), which are designed to cover the needs of 97 percent of the population, and Adequate Intakes (AI), which are used when an average nutrient requirement cannot be determined. The Patterns meet these standards for almost all nutrients. For a few nutrients (vitamin D, vitamin E, potassium, choline), amounts in the Patterns are marginal or below the RDA or AI standard for many or all age-sex groups. In most cases, an intake of these nutrients below the RDA or AI is not considered to be of public health concern. For more information on potassium and vitamin D, see Chapter 2, Underconsumed Nutrients and Nutrients of Public Health Concern.

The Healthy U.S.-Style Pattern is the base USDA Food Pattern. While the Healthy U.S.-Style Pattern is substantially unchanged from the base USDA Food Pattern of the 2010 edition of the *Dietary Guidelines*, small changes in the recommended amounts reflect updating the Patterns based on current food consumption and composition data. The Healthy U.S.-Style Pattern includes 12 calorie levels to meet the needs of individuals across the lifespan. To follow this Pattern, identify the appropriate calorie level, choose a variety of foods in each group and subgroup over time in recommended amounts, and limit choices that are not in nutrient-dense forms so that the overall calorie limit is not exceeded.

[1] For additional information and technical tables, see: U.S. Department of Agriculture. Center for Nutrition Policy and Promotion. USDA Food Patterns. Available at: http://www.cnpp.usda.gov/USDAFoodPatterns.

Table A3-1.
Healthy U.S.-Style Eating Pattern: Recommended Amounts of Food From Each Food Group at 12 Calorie Levels

Calorie Level of Pattern[a]	1,000	1,200	1,400	1,600	1,800	2,000	2,200	2,400	2,600	2,800	3,000	3,200
Food Group[b]	**Daily Amount[c]** of Food From Each Group (vegetable and protein foods subgroup amounts are per week)											
Vegetables	1 c-eq	1½ c-eq	1½ c-eq	2 c-eq	2½ c-eq	2½ c-eq	3 c-eq	3 c-eq	3½ c-eq	3½ c-eq	4 c-eq	4 c-eq
Dark-Green Vegetables (c-eq/wk)	½	1	1	1½	1½	1½	2	2	2½	2½	2½	2½
Red & Orange Vegetables (c-eq/wk)	2½	3	3	4	5½	5½	6	6	7	7	7½	7½
Legumes (Beans & Peas) (c-eq/wk)	½	½	½	1	1½	1½	2	2	2½	2½	3	3
Starchy Vegetables (c-eq/wk)	2	3½	3½	4	5	5	6	6	7	7	8	8
Other Vegetables (c-eq/wk)	1½	2½	2½	3½	4	4	5	5	5½	5½	7	7
Fruits	1 c-eq	1 c-eq	1½ c-eq	1½ c-eq	1½ c-eq	2 c-eq	2 c-eq	2 c-eq	2 c-eq	2½ c-eq	2½ c-eq	2½ c-eq
Grains	3 oz-eq	4 oz-eq	5 oz-eq	5 oz-eq	6 oz-eq	6 oz-eq	7 oz-eq	8 oz-eq	9 oz-eq	10 oz-eq	10 oz-eq	10 oz-eq
Whole Grains[d] (oz-eq/day)	1½	2	2½	3	3	3	3½	4	4½	5	5	5
Refined Grains (oz-eq/day)	1½	2	2½	2	3	3	3½	4	4½	5	5	5

Healthy U.S.-Style Eating Pattern: Recommended Amounts of Food From Each Food Group at 12 Calorie Levels

Calorie Level of Pattern[a]	1,000	1,200	1,400	1,600	1,800	2,000	2,200	2,400	2,600	2,800	3,000	3,200
Food Group[b]	Daily Amount[c] of Food From Each Group (vegetable and protein foods subgroup amounts are per week)											
Dairy	2 c-eq	2½ c-eq	2½ c-eq	3 c-eq	3 c-eq	3 c-eq	3 c-eq	3 c-eq	3 c-eq	3 c-eq	3 c-eq	3 c-eq
Protein Foods	2 oz-eq	3 oz-eq	4 oz-eq	5 oz-eq	5 oz-eq	5½ oz-eq	6 oz-eq	6½ oz-eq	6½ oz-eq	7 oz-eq	7 oz-eq	7 oz-eq
Seafood (oz-eq/wk)	3	4	6	8	8	8	9	10	10	10	10	10
Meats, Poultry, Eggs (oz-eq/wk)	10	14	19	23	23	26	28	31	31	33	33	33
Nuts Seeds, Soy Products (oz-eq/wk)	2	2	3	4	4	5	5	5	5	6	6	6
Oils	15 g	17 g	17 g	22 g	24 g	27 g	29 g	31 g	34 g	36 g	44 g	51 g
Limit on Calories for Other Uses, Calories (% of Calories)[e,f]	150 (15%)	100 (8%)	110 (8%)	130 (8%)	170 (9%)	270 (14%)	280 (13%)	350 (15%)	380 (15%)	400 (14%)	470 (16%)	610 (19%)

[a] Food intake patterns at 1,000, 1,200, and 1,400 calories are designed to meet the nutritional needs of 2- to 8-year-old children. Patterns from 1,600 to 3,200 calories are designed to meet the nutritional needs of children 9 years and older and adults. If a child 4 to 8 years of age needs more calories and, therefore, is following a pattern at 1,600 calories or more, his/her recommended amount from the dairy group should be 2.5 cups per day. Children 9 years and older and adults should not use the 1,000-, 1,200-, or 1,400-calorie patterns.

[b] Foods in each group and subgroup are:

• Vegetables

  • Dark-green vegetables: All fresh, frozen, and canned dark-green leafy vegetables and broccoli, cooked or raw: for example, broccoli; spinach; romaine; kale; collard, turnip, and mustard greens.

  • Red and orange vegetables: All fresh, frozen, and canned red and orange vegetables or juice, cooked or raw: for example, tomatoes, tomato juice, red peppers, carrots, sweet potatoes, winter squash, and pumpkin.

  • Legumes (beans and peas): All cooked from dry or canned beans and peas: for example, kidney beans, white beans, black beans, lentils, chickpeas, pinto beans, split peas, and edamame (green soybeans). Does not include green beans or green peas.

- Starchy vegetables: All fresh, frozen, and canned starchy vegetables: for example, white potatoes, corn, green peas, green lima beans, plantains, and cassava.
  - Other vegetables: All other fresh, frozen, and canned vegetables, cooked or raw: for example, iceberg lettuce, green beans, onions, cucumbers, cabbage, celery, zucchini, mushrooms, and green peppers.
- Fruits
  - All fresh, frozen, canned, and dried fruits and fruit juices: for example, oranges and orange juice, apples and apple juice, bananas, grapes, melons, berries, and raisins.
- Grains
  - Whole grains: All whole-grain products and whole grains used as ingredients: for example, whole-wheat bread, whole-grain cereals and crackers, oatmeal, quinoa, popcorn, and brown rice.
  - Refined grains: All refined-grain products and refined grains used as ingredients: for example, white breads, refined grain cereals and crackers, pasta, and white rice. Refined grain choices should be enriched.
- Dairy
  - All milk, including lactose-free and lactose-reduced products and fortified soy beverages (soymilk), yogurt, frozen yogurt, dairy desserts, and cheeses. Most choices should be fat-free or low-fat. Cream, sour cream, and cream cheese are not included due to their low calcium content.
- Protein Foods
  - All seafood, meats, poultry, eggs, soy products, nuts, and seeds. Meats and poultry should be lean or low-fat and nuts should be unsalted. Legumes (beans and peas) can be considered part of this group as well as the vegetable group, but should be counted in one group only.

[c] Food group amounts shown in cup-(c) or ounce-equivalents (oz-eq). Oils are shown in grams (g). Quantity equivalents for each food group are:

- Vegetables and fruits, 1 cup-equivalent is: 1 cup raw or cooked vegetable or fruit, 1 cup vegetable or fruit juice, 2 cups leafy salad greens, ½ cup dried fruit or vegetable.
- Grains, 1 ounce-equivalent is: ½ cup cooked rice, pasta, or cereal; 1 ounce dry pasta or rice; 1 medium (1 ounce) slice bread; 1 ounce of ready-to-eat cereal (about 1 cup of flaked cereal).
- Dairy, 1 cup-equivalent is: 1 cup milk, yogurt, or fortified soymilk; 1½ ounces natural cheese such as cheddar cheese or 2 ounces of processed cheese.
- Protein Foods, 1 ounce-equivalent is: 1 ounce lean meat, poultry, or seafood; 1 egg; ¼ cup cooked beans or tofu; 1 Tbsp peanut butter; ½ ounce nuts or seeds.

[d] Amounts of whole grains in the Patterns for children are less than the minimum of 3 oz-eq in all Patterns recommended for adults.

[e] All foods are assumed to be in nutrient-dense forms, lean or low-fat and prepared without added fats, sugars, refined starches, or salt. If all food choices to meet food group recommendations are in nutrient-dense forms, a small number of calories remain within the overall calorie limit of the Pattern (i.e., limit on calories for other uses). The number of these calories depends on the overall calorie limit in the Pattern and the amounts of food from each food group required to meet nutritional goals. Nutritional goals are higher for the 1,200- to 1,600-calorie Patterns than for the 1,000-calorie Pattern, so the limit on calories for other uses is lower in the 1,200- to 1,600-calorie Patterns. Calories up to the specified limit can be used for added sugars, added refined starches, solid fats, alcohol, or to eat more than the recommended amount of food in a food group. The overall eating Pattern also should not exceed the limits of less than 10 percent of calories from added sugars and less than 10 percent of calories from saturated fats. At most calorie levels, amounts that can be accommodated are less than these limits. For adults of legal drinking age who choose to drink alcohol, a limit of up to 1 drink per day for women and up to 2 drinks per day for men within limits on calories for other uses applies (see Appendix 9. Alcohol for additional guidance); and calories from protein, carbohydrate, and total fats should be within the Acceptable Macronutrient Distribution Ranges (AMDRs).

[f] Values are rounded.

Appendix 4.

USDA Food Patterns: Healthy Mediterranean-Style Eating Pattern

The Healthy Mediterranean-Style Pattern is adapted from the Healthy U.S.-Style Pattern, modifying amounts recommended from some food groups to more closely reflect eating patterns that have been associated with positive health outcomes in studies of Mediterranean-Style diets. Food group intakes from the studies that provided quantified data were compared to amounts in the Healthy U.S.-Style Pattern and adjustments were made to better reflect intakes of groups with Mediterranean-Style diets. The healthfulness of the Pattern was evaluated based on its similarity to food group intakes reported for groups with positive health outcomes in these studies rather than on meeting specified nutrient standards.

The Healthy Mediterranean-Style Pattern contains more fruits and seafood and less dairy than does the Healthy U.S.-Style Pattern. The changes in these amounts were limited to calorie levels appropriate for adults, because children were not part of the studies used in modifying the Pattern. The amounts of oils in the Pattern were not adjusted because the Healthy U.S.-Style Pattern already contains amounts of oils that are similar to amounts associated with positive health outcomes in the studies, and higher than typical intakes in the United States. Similarly, amounts of meat and poultry in the Healthy U.S.-Style Pattern are less than typical intakes in the United States and also similar to amounts associated with positive health outcomes in the studies.

While not evaluated on nutrient-adequacy standards, nutrient levels in the Pattern were assessed. The Pattern is similar to the Healthy U.S.-Style Pattern in nutrient content, with the exception of calcium and vitamin D. Levels of calcium and vitamin D in the Pattern are lower because less dairy is included for adults. See table footnotes for amounts of dairy recommended for children and adolescents.

To follow this Pattern, identify the appropriate calorie level, choose a variety of foods in each group and subgroup over time in recommended amounts, and limit choices that are not in nutrient-dense forms so that the overall calorie limit is not exceeded.

Table A4-1.
Healthy Mediterranean-Style Eating Pattern: Recommended Amounts of Food From Each Food Group at 12 Calorie Levels

Calorie Level of Pattern[a]	1,000	1,200	1,400	1,600	1,800	2,000	2,200	2,400	2,600	2,800	3,000	3,200
Food Group[b]	Daily Amount[c] of Food From Each Group (vegetable and protein foods subgroup amounts are per week)											
Vegetables	1 c-eq	1½ c-eq	1½ c-eq	2 c-eq	2½ c-eq	2½ c-eq	3 c-eq	3 c-eq	3½ c-eq	3½ c-eq	4 c-eq	4 c-eq
Dark-Green Vegetables (c-eq/wk)	½	1	1	1½	1½	1½	2	2	2½	2½	2½	2½
Red & Orange Vegetables (c-eq/wk)	2½	3	3	4	5½	5½	6	6	7	7	7½	7½
Legumes (Beans & Peas) (c-eq/wk)	½	½	½	1	1½	1½	2	2	2½	2½	3	3
Starchy Vegetables (c-eq/wk)	2	3½	3½	4	5	5	6	6	7	7	8	8
Other Vegetables (c-eq/wk)	1½	2½	2½	3½	4	4	5	5	5½	5½	7	7
Fruits	1 c-eq	1 c-eq	1½ c-eq	2 c-eq	2 c-eq	2½ c-eq	2½ c-eq	2½ c-eq	2½ c-eq	3 c-eq	3 c-eq	3 c-eq
Grains	3 oz-eq	4 oz-eq	5 oz-eq	5 oz-eq	6 oz-eq	6 oz-eq	7 oz-eq	8 oz-eq	9 oz-eq	10 oz-eq	10 oz-eq	10 oz-eq
Whole Grains[d] (oz-eq/day)	1½	2	2½	3	3	3	3½	4	4½	5	5	5
Refined Grains (oz-eq/day)	1½	2	2½	2	3	3	3½	4	4½	5	5	5

Table A4-1. *(continued...)*

Healthy Mediterranean-Style Eating Pattern: Recommended Amounts of Food From Each Food Group at 12 Calorie Levels

Calorie Level of Pattern[a]	1,000	1,200	1,400	1,600	1,800	2,000	2,200	2,400	2,600	2,800	3,000	3,200
Food Group[b]	Daily Amount[c] of Food From Each Group (vegetable and protein foods subgroup amounts are per week)											
Dairy[e]	2 c-eq	2½ c-eq	2½ c-eq	2 c-eq	2 c-eq	2 c-eq	2 c-eq	2½ c-eq	2½ c-eq	2½ c-eq	2½ c-eq	2½ c-eq
Protein Foods	2 oz-eq	3 oz-eq	4 oz-eq	5½ oz-eq	6 oz-eq	6½ oz-eq	7 oz-eq	7½ oz-eq	7½ oz-eq	8 oz-eq	8 oz-eq	8 oz-eq
Seafood (oz-eq/wk)[f]	3	4	6	11	15	15	16	16	17	17	17	17
Meats, Poultry, Eggs (oz-eq/wk)	10	14	19	23	23	26	28	31	31	33	33	33
Nuts Seeds, Soy Products (oz-eq/wk)	2	2	3	4	4	5	5	5	5	6	6	6
Oils	15 g	17 g	17 g	22 g	24 g	27 g	29 g	31 g	34 g	36 g	44 g	51 g
Limit on Calories for Other Uses, Calories (% of Calories)[g,h]	150 (15%)	100 (8%)	110 (8%)	140 (9%)	160 (9%)	260 (13%)	270 (12%)	300 (13%)	330 (13%)	350 (13%)	430 (14%)	570 (18%)

[a, b, c, d] See Appendix 3. USDA Food Patterns: Healthy U.S.-Style Eating Pattern, notes a through d.

[e] Amounts of dairy recommended for children and adolescents are as follows, regardless of the calorie level of the Pattern: For 2 year-olds, 2 cup-eq per day; for 3 to 8 year-olds, 2 ½ cup-eq per day; for 9 to 18 year-olds, 3 cup-eq per day.

[f] The U.S. Food and Drug Administration (FDA) and the U.S. Environmental Protection Agency (EPA) provide joint guidance regarding seafood consumption for women who are pregnant or breastfeeding and young children. For more information, see the FDA or EPA websites www.FDA.gov/fishadvice; www.EPA.gov/fishadvice.

[g,h] See Appendix 3, notes e through f.

Appendix 5.

USDA Food Patterns: Healthy Vegetarian Eating Pattern

The Healthy Vegetarian Pattern is adapted from the Healthy U.S.-Style Pattern, modifying amounts recommended from some food groups to more closely reflect eating patterns reported by self-identified vegetarians in the National Health and Nutrition Examination Survey (NHANES). This analysis allowed development of a Pattern that is based on evidence of the foods and amounts consumed by vegetarians, in addition to meeting the same nutrient and Dietary Guidelines standards as the Healthy U.S.-Style Pattern. Based on a comparison of the food choices of these vegetarians to nonvegetarians in NHANES, amounts of soy products (particularly tofu and

other processed soy products), legumes, nuts and seeds, and whole grains were increased, and meat, poultry, and seafood were eliminated. Dairy and eggs were included because they were consumed by the majority of these vegetarians. This Pattern can be vegan if all dairy choices are comprised of fortified soy beverages (soymilk) or other plant-based dairy substitutes. Note that vegetarian adaptations of the USDA Food Patterns were included in the *2010 Dietary Guidelines*. However, those adaptations did not modify the underlying structure of the Patterns, but substituted the same amounts of plant foods for animal foods in each food group. In contrast, the current

Healthy Vegetarian Pattern includes changes in food group composition and amounts, based on assessing the food choices of vegetarians. The Pattern is similar in meeting nutrient standards to the Healthy U.S.-Style Pattern, but somewhat higher in calcium and fiber and lower in vitamin D due to differences in the foods included.

To follow this Pattern, identify the appropriate calorie level, choose a variety of foods in each group and subgroup over time in recommended amounts, and limit choices that are not in nutrient-dense forms so that the overall calorie limit is not exceeded.

Table A5-1.

Healthy Vegetarian Eating Pattern: Recommended Amounts of Food From Each Food Group at 12 Calorie Levels

Calorie Level of Pattern[a]	1,000	1,200	1,400	1,600	1,800	2,000	2,200	2,400	2,600	2,800	3,000	3,200
Food Group[b]	Daily Amount[c] of Food From Each Group (vegetable and protein foods subgroup amounts are per week)											
Vegetables	1 c-eq	1½ c-eq	1½ c-eq	2 c-eq	2½ c-eq	2½ c-eq	3 c-eq	3 c-eq	3½ c-eq	3½ c-eq	4 c-eq	4 c-eq
Dark-Green Vegetables (c-eq/wk)	½	1	1	1½	1½	1½	2	2	2½	2½	2½	2½
Red & Orange Vegetables (c-eq/wk)	2½	3	3	4	5½	5½	6	6	7	7	7½	7½
Legumes (Beans & Peas) (c-eq/wk)[d]	½	½	½	1	1½	1½	2	2	2½	2½	3	3
Starchy Vegetables (c-eq/wk)	2	3½	3½	4	5	5	6	6	7	7	8	8
Other Vegetables (c-eq/wk)	1½	2½	2½	3½	4	4	5	5	5½	5½	7	7
Fruits	1 c-eq	1 c-eq	1½ c-eq	1½ c-eq	1½ c-eq	2 c-eq	2 c-eq	2 c-eq	2 c-eq	2½ c-eq	2½ c-eq	2½ c-eq
Grains	3 oz-eq	4 oz-eq	5 oz-eq	5½ oz-eq	6½ oz-eq	6½ oz-eq	7½ oz-eq	8½ oz-eq	9½ oz-eq	10½ oz-eq	10½ oz-eq	10½ oz-eq
Whole Grains[e] (oz-eq/day)	1½	2	2½	3	3½	3½	4	4½	5	5½	5½	5½
Refined Grains (oz-eq/day)	1½	2	2½	2½	3	3	3 ½	4	4 ½	5	5	5
Dairy	2 c-eq	2.5 c-eq	2.5 c-eq	3 c-eq	3 c-eq	3 c-eq	3 c-eq	3 c-eq	3 c-eq	3 c-eq	3 c-eq	3 c-eq

Calorie Level of Pattern[a]	1,000	1,200	1,400	1,600	1,800	2,000	2,200	2,400	2,600	2,800	3,000	3,200
Food Group[b]	Daily Amount[c] of Food From Each Group (vegetable and protein foods subgroup amounts are per week)											
Protein Foods	1 oz-eq	1½ oz-eq	2 oz-eq	2½ oz-eq	3 oz-eq	3½ oz-eq	3½ oz-eq	4 oz-eq	4½ oz-eq	5 oz-eq	5½ oz-eq	6 oz-eq
Eggs (oz-eq/wk)	2	3	3	3	3	3	3	3	3	4	4	4
Legumes (Beans & Peas) (oz-eq/wk)[d]	1	2	4	4	6	6	6	8	9	10	11	12
Soy Products (oz-eq/wk)	2	3	4	6	6	8	8	9	10	11	12	13
Nuts & Seeds (oz-eq/wk)	2	2	3	5	6	7	7	8	9	10	12	13
Oils	15 g	17 g	17 g	22 g	24 g	27 g	29 g	31 g	34 g	36 g	44 g	51 g
Limit on Calories for Other Uses, Calories (% of Calories)[f,g]	190 (19%)	170 (14%)	190 (14%)	180 (11%)	190 (11%)	290 (15%)	330 (15%)	390 (16%)	390 (15%)	400 (14%)	440 (15%)	550 (17%)

[a, b, c] See Appendix 3. USDA Food Patterns: Healthy U.S.-Style Eating Pattern, notes a through c.

[d] About half of total legumes are shown as vegetables, in cup-eq, and half as protein foods, in oz-eq. Total legumes in the Patterns, in cup-eq, is the amount in the vegetable group plus the amount in protein foods group (in oz-eq) divided by 4:

Calorie Level of Pattern[a]	1,000	1,200	1,400	1,600	1,800	2,000	2,200	2,400	2,600	2,800	3,000	3,200
Total Legumes (Beans & Peas) (c-eq/wk)	1	1	1½	2	3	3	3½	4	5	5	6	6

[e, f, g] See Appendix 3, notes d through f.

Appendix 6.
Glossary of Terms

A

Acculturation—The process by which individuals who immigrate into a new country adopt the attitudes, values, customs, beliefs, and behaviors of the new culture. Acculturation is the gradual exchange between the original attitudes and behaviors associated with the originating country and those of the host culture.

Added Refined Starch—The starch constituent (see Carbohydrates) of a grain, such as corn, or of a vegetable, such as potato, used as an ingredient in another food. Starches have been refined to remove other components of the food, such as fiber, protein, and minerals. Refined starches can be added to foods as a thickener, a stabilizer, a bulking agent, or an anti-caking agent. While refined starches are made from grains or vegetables, they contain little or none of the many other components of these foods that together create a nutrient-dense food. They are a source of calories but few or no other nutrients.

Added Sugars—Syrups and other caloric sweeteners used as a sweetener in other food products. Naturally occurring sugars such as those in fruit or milk are not added sugars. Specific examples of added sugars that can be listed as an ingredient include brown sugar, corn sweetener, corn syrup, dextrose, fructose, glucose, high-fructose corn syrup, honey, invert sugar, lactose, malt syrup, maltose, molasses, raw sugar, sucrose, trehalose, and turbinado sugar. (See Carbohydrates, Sugars.)

B

Body Mass Index (BMI)—A measure of weight in kilograms (kg) relative to height in meters squared (m^2). BMI is considered a reasonably reliable indicator of total body fat, which is related to the risk of disease and death. BMI status categories include underweight, healthy weight, overweight, and obese (**Table A6-1**). Overweight and obese describe ranges of weight that are greater than what is considered healthy

Table A6-1.
Body Mass Index (BMI) & Corresponding Body Weight Categories for Children & Adults

Body Weight Category	Children & Adolescents (Ages 2 to 19 Years) (BMI-for-Age Percentile Range)	Adults (BMI)
Underweight	Less than the 5th percentile	Less than 18.5 kg/m^2
Normal Weight	5th percentile to less than the 85th percentile	18.5 to 24.9 kg/m^2
Overweight	85th to less than the 95th percentile	25.0 to 29.9 kg/m^2
Obese	Equal to or greater than the 95th percentile	30.0 kg/m^2 & greater

for a given height, while underweight describes a weight that is lower than what is considered healthy. Because children and adolescents are growing, their BMI is plotted on growth charts for sex and age. The percentile indicates the relative position of the child's BMI among children of the same sex and age.

C

Calorie Balance—The balance between calories consumed through eating and drinking and calories expended through physical activity and metabolic processes.

- **Calorie**—A unit commonly used to measure energy content of foods and beverages as well as energy use (expenditure) by the body. A kilocalorie is equal to the amount of energy (heat) required to raise the temperature of 1 kilogram of water 1 degree centigrade. Energy is required to sustain the body's various functions, including metabolic processes and physical activity. Carbohydrate, fat, protein, and alcohol provide all of the energy supplied by foods and beverages. If not specified explicitly, references to "calories" refer to "kilocalories."

Carbohydrates—One of the macronutrients and a source of energy. They include sugars, starches, and fiber:

- **Fiber**—Total fiber is the sum of *dietary fiber* and *functional fiber*. Dietary fiber consists of nondigestible carbohydrates and lignin that are intrinsic and intact in plants (i.e., the fiber naturally occurring in foods). Functional fiber consists of isolated, nondigestible carbohydrates that have beneficial physiological effects in humans. Functional fibers are either extracted from natural sources or are synthetically manufactured and added to foods, beverages, and supplements.

- **Starches**—Many glucose units linked together into long chains. Examples of foods containing starch include vegetables (e.g., potatoes, carrots), grains (e.g., brown rice, oats, wheat, barley, corn), and legumes (beans and peas; e.g., kidney beans, garbanzo beans, lentils, split peas).

- **Sugars**—Composed of one unit (a monosaccharide, such as glucose or fructose) or two joined units (a disaccharide, such as lactose or sucrose). Sugars include those occurring naturally in foods and beverages, those added to foods and beverages during processing and preparation, and those consumed separately. (See Added Sugars.)

Cardiovascular Disease (CVD)—Heart disease as well as diseases of the blood vessel system (arteries, capillaries, veins) that can lead to heart attack, chest pain (angina), or stroke.

Cholesterol—A natural sterol present in all animal tissues. Free cholesterol is a component of cell membranes and serves as a precursor for steroid hormones (estrogen, testosterone, aldosterone), and for bile acids. Humans are able to synthesize sufficient cholesterol to meet biologic requirements, and there is no evidence for a dietary requirement for cholesterol.

- **Blood Cholesterol**—Cholesterol that travels in the serum of the blood as distinct particles containing both lipids and proteins (lipoproteins). Also referred to as serum cholesterol. Two kinds of lipoproteins are:

  - **High-Density Lipoprotein (HDL-cholesterol)**—Blood cholesterol often called "good" cholesterol; carries cholesterol from tissues to the liver, which removes it from the body.

  - **Low-Density Lipoprotein (LDL-Cholesterol)**—Blood cholesterol often called "bad" cholesterol; carries cholesterol to arteries and tissues. A high LDL-cholesterol level in the blood leads to a buildup of cholesterol in arteries.

- **Dietary Cholesterol**—Cholesterol found in foods of animal origin, including meat, seafood, poultry, eggs, and dairy products. Plant foods, such as grains, vegetables, fruits, and oils do not contain dietary cholesterol.

Cup-Equivalent (cup-eq or c-eq)—The amount of a food or beverage product that is considered equal to 1 cup from the vegetables, fruits, or dairy food groups. A cup-eq for some foods or beverages may differ from a measured cup in volume because the foods have been concentrated (such as raisins or tomato paste), the foods are airy in their raw form and do not compress well into a cup (such as salad greens), or the foods are measured in a different form (such as cheese).

D

DASH Eating Plan—The DASH (Dietary Approaches to Stop Hypertension) Eating Plan exemplifies healthy eating. It was designed to increase intake of foods expected to lower blood pressure while being heart healthy and meeting Institute of Medicine (IOM) nutrient recommendations. It is available at specific calorie levels. It was adapted from the dietary pattern developed for the Dietary Approaches to Stop Hypertension (DASH) research trials. In the trials, the DASH dietary pattern lowered blood pressure and LDL-cholesterol levels, resulting in reduced cardiovascular disease risk. The DASH Eating Plan is low in saturated fats and rich in potassium, calcium, and magnesium, as well as fiber and protein. It also is lower in sodium than the typical American diet, and includes menus with two levels of sodium, 2,300 and 1,500 mg per day. It meets the Dietary Reference Intakes for all essential nutrients and stays within limits for overconsumed nutrients, while allowing adaptable food choices based on food preferences, cost, and availability.

Diabetes—A disorder of metabolism—the way the body uses digested food (specifically carbohydrate) for growth and energy. In diabetes, the pancreas either produces little or no insulin (a hormone that helps glucose, the body's main source of fuel, get into cells), or the cells do not respond appropriately to the insulin that is produced, which causes too much glucose to be released in the blood. The three main types of diabetes are type 1, type 2, and gestational diabetes. If not controlled, diabetes can lead to serious complications.

Dietary Reference Intakes (DRIs)—A set of nutrient-based reference values that are quantitative estimates of nutrient intakes to be used for planning and assessing diets for healthy people. DRIs expand on the periodic reports called Recommended Dietary Allowances (RDAs), which were first published by the Institute of Medicine in 1941.

- **Acceptable Macronutrient Distribution Ranges (AMDR)**—Range of intake for a particular energy source (i.e., carbohydrate, fat, and protein) that is associated with reduced risk of chronic disease while providing intakes of essential nutrients. If an individual's intake is outside of the AMDR, there is a potential of increasing the risk of chronic diseases and/or insufficient intakes of essential nutrients.

- **Adequate Intakes (AI)**—A recommended average daily nutrient intake level based on observed or experimentally determined approximations or estimates of mean nutrient intake by a group (or groups) of apparently healthy people. An AI is used when the Recommended Dietary Allowance cannot be determined.

- **Estimated Average Requirements (EAR)**—The average daily nutrient intake level estimated to meet the requirement of half the healthy individuals in a particular life stage and sex group.

- **Recommended Dietary Allowances (RDA)**—The average daily dietary intake level that is sufficient to meet the nutrient requirement of nearly all (97 to 98%) healthy individuals in a particular life stage and sex group.

- **Tolerable Upper Intake Levels (UL)**—The highest average daily nutrient intake level likely to pose no risk of adverse health effects for nearly all individuals in a particular life stage and sex group. As intake increases above the UL, the potential risk of adverse health effects increases.

E

Eating Behaviors—Individual behaviors that affect food and beverage choices and intake patterns, such as what, where, when, why, and how much people eat.

Eating Pattern (also called "dietary pattern")—The combination of foods and beverages that constitute an individual's complete dietary intake over time. This may be a description of a customary way of eating or a description of a combination of foods recommended for consumption. Specific examples include USDA Food Patterns and the Dietary Approaches to Stop Hypertension (DASH) Eating Plan. (See USDA Food Patterns and DASH Eating Plan.)

Energy Drink—A beverage that contains caffeine as an ingredient, along with other ingredients, such as taurine, herbal supplements, vitamins, and added sugars. It is usually marketed as a product that can improve perceived energy, stamina, athletic performance, or concentration.

Enrichment—The addition of specific nutrients (i.e., iron, thiamin, riboflavin, and niacin) to refined grain products in order to replace losses of the nutrients that occur during processing. Enrichment of refined grains is not mandatory; however, those that are labeled as enriched (e.g., enriched flour) must meet the standard of identity for enrichment set by the FDA. When cereal grains are labeled as enriched, it is mandatory that they be fortified with folic acid. (The addition of specific nutrients to whole-grain products is referred to as fortification; see Fortification.)

Essential Nutrient—A vitamin, mineral, fatty acid, or amino acid required for normal body functioning that either cannot be synthesized by the body at all, or cannot be synthesized in amounts adequate for good health, and thus must be obtained from a dietary source. Other food components, such as dietary fiber, while not essential, also are considered to be nutrients.

Existing Report—An existing systematic review, meta-analysis, or report by a Federal agency or leading scientific organization examined by the 2015 Dietary Guidelines Advisory Committee in its review of the scientific evidence. A systematic process was used by the Advisory Committee to assess the quality and comprehensiveness of the review for addressing the question of interest. (See Nutrition Evidence Library (NEL) systematic review.)

F

Fats—One of the macronutrients and a source of energy. (See Solid Fats and Oils.)

- **Monounsaturated Fatty Acids (MUFAs)**—Fatty acids that have one double bond and are usually liquid at room temperature. Plant sources rich in MUFAs include vegetable oils (e.g., canola, olive, high oleic safflower and sunflower), as well as nuts.

- **Polyunsaturated Fatty Acids (PUFAs)**—Fatty acids that have two or more double bonds and are usually liquid at room temperature. Primary sources are vegetable oils and some nuts and seeds. PUFAs provide essential fats such as n-3 and n-6 fatty acids.

- **n-3 PUFAs**—A carboxylic acid with an 18-carbon chain and three cis double bonds, Alpha-linolenic acid (ALA) is an n-3 fatty acid that is essential in the diet because it cannot be synthesized by humans. Primary sources include soybean oil, canola oil, walnuts, and flaxseed. Eicosapentaenoic acid (EPA) and docosahexaenoic acid (DHA) are very long chain n-3 fatty acids that are contained in fish and shellfish. Also called omega-3 fatty acids.

- **n-6 PUFAs**—A carboxylic acid with an 18-carbon chain and two cis double bonds, Linoleic acid (LA), one of the n-6 fatty acids, is essential in the diet because it cannot be synthesized by humans. Primary sources are nuts and liquid vegetable oils, including soybean oil, corn oil, and safflower oil. Also called omega-6 fatty acids.

- **Saturated Fatty Acids**—Fatty acids that have no double bonds. Fats high in saturated fatty acids are usually solid at room temperature. Major sources include animal products such as meats and dairy products, and tropical oils such as coconut or palm oils.

- **Trans Fatty Acids**—Unsaturated fatty acids that are structurally different from the unsaturated fatty acids that occur naturally in plant foods. Sources of trans fatty acids include partially hydrogenated vegetable oils used in processed foods such as desserts, microwave popcorn, frozen pizza, some margarines, and coffee creamer. Trans fatty acids also are present naturally in foods that come from ruminant animals (e.g., cattle and sheep), such as dairy products, beef, and lamb.

Food Access—Ability to obtain and maintain levels of sufficient amounts of healthy, safe, and affordable food for all family members in various settings including where they live, learn, work and play. Food access is often measured by distance to a store or the number of stores in an area; individual-level resources such as family income or vehicle availability; and neighborhood-level indicators of resources, such as average income of the neighborhood and the availability of public transportation.

Food Categories—A method of grouping similar foods in their as-consumed forms, for descriptive purposes. The USDA's Agricultural Research Service (ARS) has created 150 mutually exclusive food categories to account for each food or beverage item reported in What We Eat in America (WWEIA), the food intake survey component of the National Health and Nutrition Examination Survey (for more information, visit: http://seprl.ars.usda.gov/Services/docs.htm?docid=23429). Examples of WWEIA Food Categories include soups, nachos, and yeast breads. In contrast to food groups, items are not disaggregated into their component parts for assignment to food categories. For example, all pizzas are put into the pizza category.

Food Hub—A community space anchored by a food store with adjacent social and financial services where businesses or organizations can actively manage the aggregation, distribution, and marketing of source-identified food products to strengthen their ability to satisfy wholesale, retail, and institutional demand.

Food Groups—A method of grouping similar foods for descriptive and guidance purposes. Food groups in the USDA Food Patterns are defined as vegetables, fruits, grains, dairy, and protein foods. Some of these groups are divided into subgroups, such as dark-green vegetables or whole grains, which may have intake goals or limits. Foods are grouped within food groups based on their similarity in nutritional composition and other dietary benefits. For assignment to food groups, mixed dishes are disaggregated into their major component parts.

Food Pattern Modeling—The process of developing and adjusting daily intake amounts from food categories or groups to meet specific criteria, such as meeting nutrient intake goals, limiting nutrients or other food components, or varying proportions or amounts of specific food categories or groups. This methodology includes using current food consumption data to determine the mix and proportions of foods to include in each group, using current food composition data to select a nutrient-dense representative for each food, calculating nutrient profiles for each food group using these nutrient-dense representative foods, and modeling various combinations of foods and amounts to meet specific criteria. (See USDA Food Patterns.)

Food & Nutrition Policies—Regulations, laws, policymaking actions, or formal or informal rules established by formal organizations or government units. Food and nutrition policies are those that influence food settings and/or eating behaviors to improve food and/or nutrition choices, and potentially, health outcomes (e.g., body weight).

Fortification—As defined by the U.S. Food and Drug Administration (FDA), the deliberate addition of one or more essential nutrients to a food, whether or not it is normally contained in the food. Fortification may be used to prevent or correct a demonstrated deficiency in the population or specific population groups; restore naturally occurring nutrients lost during processing, storage, or handling; or to add a nutrient to a food at the level found in a comparable traditional food. When cereal grains are labeled as enriched, it is mandatory that they be fortified with folic acid.

H

Health—A state of complete physical, mental, and social well-being and not merely the absence of disease or infirmity.

Healthy Eating Index (HEI)—A measure of diet quality that assesses adherence to the *Dietary Guidelines*. The HEI is used to monitor diet quality in the United States and to examine relationships between diet and health-related outcomes. The HEI is a scoring metric that can be applied to any defined set of foods, such as previously collected dietary data, a defined menu, or a market basket. Thus, the HEI can be used to assess the quality of food assistance packages, menus, and the U.S. food supply.

High-Intensity Sweeteners—Ingredients commonly used as sugar substitutes or sugar alternatives to sweeten and enhance the flavor of foods and beverages. People may choose these sweeteners in place of sugar for a number of reasons, including that they contribute few or no calories to the diet. Because high-intensity sweeteners are many times sweeter than table sugar (sucrose), smaller amounts of high-intensity sweeteners are needed to achieve the same level of sweetness as sugar in food and beverages. (Other terms commonly used to refer to sugar substitutes or alternatives include non-caloric, low-calorie, no-calorie, and artificial sweeteners, which may have different definitions and applications. A high-intensity sweetener may or may not be non-caloric, low-calorie, no-calorie, or artificial sweeteners.)

Household Food Insecurity—Circumstances in which the availability of nutritionally adequate and safe food, or the ability to acquire acceptable foods in socially acceptable ways, is limited or uncertain.

Hypertension—A condition, also known as high blood pressure, in which blood pressure remains elevated over time. Hypertension makes the heart work too hard, and the high force of the blood flow can harm arteries and organs, such as the heart, kidneys, brain, and eyes. Uncontrolled hypertension can lead to heart attacks, heart failure, kidney disease, stroke, and blindness. Prehypertension is defined as blood pressure that is higher than normal but not high enough to be defined as hypertension.

M

Macronutrient—A dietary component that provides energy. Macronutrients include protein, fats, carbohydrates, and alcohol.

Meats & Poultry—Foods that come from the flesh of land animals and birds. In the USDA Food Patterns, organs (such as liver) are also considered to be meat or poultry.

- **Meat** (also known as "red meat")—All forms of beef, pork, lamb, veal, goat, and non-bird game (e.g., venison, bison, elk).

- **Poultry**—All forms of chicken, turkey, duck, geese, guineas, and game birds (e.g., quail, pheasant).

- **Lean Meat & Lean Poultry**—Any meat or poultry that contains less than 10 g of fat, 4.5 g or less of saturated fats, and less than 95 mg of cholesterol per 100 g and per labeled serving size, based on USDA definitions for food label use. Examples include 95% lean cooked ground beef, beef top round steak or roast, beef tenderloin, pork top loin chop or roast, pork tenderloin, ham or turkey deli slices, skinless chicken breast, and skinless turkey breast.

- **Processed Meat & Processed Poultry**—All meat or poultry products preserved by smoking, curing, salting, and/or the addition of chemical preservatives. Processed meats and poultry include all types of meat or poultry sausages (bologna, frankfurters, luncheon meats and loaves, sandwich spreads, viennas, chorizos, kielbasa, pepperoni, salami, and summer sausages), bacon, smoked or cured ham or pork shoulder, corned beef, pastrami, pig's feet, beef jerky, marinated chicken breasts, and smoked turkey products.

Mixed Dishes—Savory food items eaten as a single entity that include foods from more than one food group. These foods often are mixtures of grains, protein foods, vegetables, and/or dairy. Examples of mixed dishes include burgers, sandwiches, tacos, burritos, pizzas, macaroni and cheese, stir-fries, spaghetti and meatballs, casseroles, soups, egg rolls, and Caesar salad.

Moderate Alcohol Consumption—Up to one drink per day for women and up to two drinks per day for men. One drink-equivalent is described using the reference beverages of 12 fl oz of regular beer (5% alcohol), 5 fl oz of wine (12% alcohol), or 1.5 fl oz of 80 proof (40%) distilled spirits. One drink-equivalent is described as containing 14 g (0.6 fl oz) of pure alcohol.[1]

Multi-Component Intervention—Interventions that use a combination of strategies to promote behavior change. These strategies can be employed across or within different settings or levels of influence.

Multi-Level Intervention—Interventions are those that target change at the individual level as well as additional levels, such as in the community (e.g., public health campaigns), schools (e.g., education), and food service (e.g., menu modification).

N

Nutrient Dense—A characteristic of foods and beverages that provide vitamins, minerals, and other substances that contribute to adequate nutrient intakes or may have positive health effects, with little or no solid fats and added sugars, refined starches, and sodium. Ideally, these foods and beverages also are in forms that retain naturally occurring components, such as dietary fiber. All vegetables, fruits, whole grains, seafood, eggs, beans and peas, unsalted nuts and seeds, fat-free and low-fat dairy products, and lean meats and poultry—when prepared with little or no added solid fats, sugars, refined starches, and sodium—are nutrient-dense foods. These foods contribute to meeting food group recommendations within calorie and sodium limits. The term "nutrient dense" indicates the nutrients and other beneficial substances in a food have not been "diluted" by the addition of calories from added solid fats, sugars, or refined starches, or by the

solid fats naturally present in the food.

Nutrient of Concern—Nutrients that are overconsumed or underconsumed and current intakes may pose a substantial public health concern. Data on nutrient intake, corroborated with biochemical markers of nutritional status where available, and association with health outcomes are all used to establish a nutrient as a nutrient of concern. Underconsumed nutrients, or "shortfall nutrients," are those with a high prevalence of inadequate intake either across the U.S. population or in specific groups, relative to IOM-based standards, such as the Estimated Average Requirement (EAR) or the Adequate Intake (AI). Overconsumed nutrients are those with a high prevalence of excess intake either across the population or in specific groups, related to IOM-based standards such as the Tolerable Upper Intake Level (UL) or other expert group standards.

Nutrition Evidence Library (NEL) Systematic Review—A process that uses state-of-the-art methods to identify, evaluate, and synthesize research to provide timely answers to important food and nutrition-related questions to inform U.S. Federal nutrition policies, programs, and recommendations. This rigorous, protocol-driven methodology is designed to minimize bias, maximize transparency, and ensure the use of all available relevant and high-quality research. The NEL is a program within the USDA Center for Nutrition Policy and Promotion. For more detailed information, visit: www.NEL.gov.

O

Oils—Fats that are liquid at room temperature. Oils come from many different plants and some fish. Some common oils include canola, corn, olive, peanut, safflower, soybean, and sunflower oils.

A number of foods are naturally high in oils such as nuts, olives, some fish, and avocados. Foods that are mainly made up of oil include mayonnaise, certain salad dressings, and soft (tub or squeeze) margarine with no *trans* fats. Oils are high in monounsaturated or polyunsaturated fats, and lower in saturated fats than solid fats. A few plant oils, termed tropical oils, including coconut oil, palm oil and palm kernel oil, are high in saturated fats and for nutritional purposes should be considered as solid fats. Partially hydrogenated oils that contain *trans* fats should also be considered as solid fats for nutritional purposes. (See Fats.)

Ounce-Equivalent (oz-eq)—The amount of a food product that is considered equal to 1 ounce from the grain or protein foods food group. An oz-eq for some foods may be less than a measured ounce in weight if the food is concentrated or low in water content (nuts, peanut butter, dried meats, flour) or more than a measured ounce in weight if the food contains a large amount of water (tofu, cooked beans, cooked rice or pasta).

P

Physical Activity—Any bodily movement produced by the contraction of skeletal muscle that increases energy expenditure above a basal level; generally refers to the subset of physical activity that enhances health.

Point-of-Purchase—A place where sales are made. Various intervention strategies have been proposed to affect individuals' purchasing decisions at the point of purchase, such as board or menu labeling with various amounts of nutrition information or shelf tags in grocery stores.

Portion Size—The amount of a food served or consumed in one eating

---

[1] Drink-equivalents are not intended to serve as a standard drink definition for regulatory purposes.

occasion. A portion is not a standardized amount, and the amount considered to be a portion is subjective and varies.

Prehypertension—See Hypertension.

Protein—One of the macronutrients; a major functional and structural component of every animal cell. Proteins are composed of amino acids, nine of which are indispensable (essential), meaning they cannot be synthesized by humans and therefore must be obtained from the diet. The quality of dietary protein is determined by its amino acid profile relative to human requirements as determined by the body's requirements for growth, maintenance, and repair. Protein quality is determined by two factors: digestibility and amino acid composition.

R

Refined Grains—Grains and grain products with the bran and germ removed; any grain product that is not a whole-grain product. Many refined grains are low in fiber but enriched with thiamin, riboflavin, niacin, and iron, and fortified with folic acid.

S

Screen Time—Time spent in front of a computer, television, video or computer game system, smart phone or tablet, or related device.

Seafood—Marine animals that live in the sea and in freshwater lakes and rivers. Seafood includes fish (e.g., salmon, tuna, trout, and tilapia) and shellfish (e.g., shrimp, crab, and oysters).

Sedentary Behavior—Any waking activity predominantly done while in a sitting or reclining posture. A behavior that expends energy at or minimally above a person's resting level (between 1.0 and 1.5 metabolic equivalents) is considered sedentary behavior.

Serving Size—A standardized amount of a food, such as a cup or an ounce, used in providing information about a food within a food group, such as in dietary guidance. Serving size on the Nutrition Facts label is determined based on the Reference Amounts Customarily Consumed (RACC) for foods that have similar dietary usage, product characteristics, and customarily consumed amounts for consumers to make "like product" comparisons. (See Portion Size.)

Shortfall Nutrient— See Nutrient of Concern.

Social-Ecological Model— A framework developed to illustrate how sectors, settings, social and cultural norms, and individual factors converge to influence individual food and physical activity choices.

Solid Fats—Fats that are usually not liquid at room temperature. Solid fats are found in animal foods, except for seafood, and can be made from vegetable oils through hydrogenation. Some tropical oil plants, such as coconut and palm, are considered as solid fats due to their fatty acid composition. The fat component of milk and cream (butter) is solid at room temperature. Solid fats contain more saturated fats and/or *trans* fats than liquid oils (e.g., soybean, canola, and corn oils), with lower amounts of monounsaturated or polyunsaturated fatty acids. Common fats considered to be solid fats include: butter, beef fat (tallow), chicken fat, pork fat (lard), shortening, coconut oil, palm oil and palm kernel oil. Foods high in solid fats include: full-fat (regular) cheeses, creams, whole milk, ice cream, marbled cuts of meats, regular ground beef, bacon, sausages, poultry skin, and many baked goods made with solid fats (such as cookies, crackers, doughnuts, pastries, and croissants). (See Fats and Nutrient Dense)

Sugar-Sweetened Beverages— Liquids that are sweetened with various forms of added sugars. These beverages include, but are not limited to, soda (regular, not sugar-free), fruitades, sports drinks, energy drinks, sweetened waters, and coffee and tea beverages with added sugars. Also called calorically sweetened beverages. (See Added Sugars and Carbohydrates: Sugars.)

U

USDA Food Patterns—A set of eating patterns that exemplify healthy eating, which all include recommended intakes for the five food groups (vegetables, fruits, grains, dairy, and protein foods) and for subgroups within the vegetables, grains, and protein foods groups. They also recommend an allowance for intake of oils. Patterns are provided at 12 calorie levels from 1,000 to 3,200 calories to meet varied calorie needs. The Healthy U.S.-Style Pattern is the base USDA Food Pattern.

- **Healthy U.S.-Style Eating Pattern**—A pattern that exemplifies healthy eating based on the types and proportions of foods Americans typically consume, but in nutrient-dense forms and appropriate amounts, designed to meet nutrient needs while not exceeding calorie requirements. It is substantially unchanged from the primary USDA Food Patterns of the *2010 Dietary Guidelines*. This pattern is evaluated in comparison to meeting Dietary Reference Intakes for essential nutrients and staying within limits set by the IOM or *Dietary Guidelines* for overconsumed food components. It aligns closely with the Dietary Approaches to Stop Hypertension

(DASH) Eating Plan, a guide for healthy eating based on the DASH diet which was tested in clinical trials. (See Nutrient Dense and DASH Eating Plan.)

- **Healthy Mediterranean-Style Eating Pattern**—A pattern that exemplifies healthy eating, designed by modifying the Healthy U.S.-Style Pattern to more closely reflect eating patterns that have been associated with positive health outcomes in studies of Mediterranean-Style diets. This pattern is evaluated based on its similarity to food group intakes of groups with positive health outcomes in these studies rather than on meeting specified nutrient standards. It differs from the Healthy U.S.-Style Pattern in that it includes more fruits and seafood and less dairy.

- **Healthy Vegetarian Eating Pattern**—A pattern that exemplifies healthy eating, designed by modifying the Healthy U.S.-Style Pattern to more closely reflect eating patterns reported by self-identified vegetarians. This pattern is evaluated in comparison to meeting Dietary Reference Intakes for essential nutrients and staying within limits set by the IOM or *Dietary Guidelines* for overconsumed food components. It differs from the Healthy U.S.-Style Pattern in that it includes more legumes, soy products, nuts and seeds, and whole grains, and no meat, poultry, or seafood.

V

Variety—A diverse assortment of foods and beverages across and within all food groups and subgroups selected to fulfill the recommended amounts without exceeding the limits for calories and other dietary components. For example, in the vegetables food group, selecting a variety of foods could be accomplished over the course of a week by choosing from all subgroups, including dark green, red and orange, legumes (beans and peas), starchy, and other vegetables.

W

Whole Fruits—All fresh, frozen, canned, and dried fruit but not fruit juice.

Whole Grains—Grains and grain products made from the entire grain seed, usually called the kernel, which consists of the bran, germ, and endosperm. If the kernel has been cracked, crushed, or flaked, it must retain the same relative proportions of bran, germ, and endosperm as the original grain in order to be called whole grain. Many, but not all, whole grains are also sources of dietary fiber.

Appendix 7.

Nutritional Goals for Age-Sex Groups Based on Dietary Reference Intakes & *Dietary Guidelines* Recommendations

Table A7-1.

Daily Nutritional Goals for Age-Sex Groups Based on Dietary Reference Intakes & *Dietary Guidelines* Recommendations

	Source of Goal[a]	Child 1-3	Female 4-8	Male 4-8	Female 9-13	Male 9-13	Female 14-18	Male 14-18	Female 19-30	Male 19-30	Female 31-50	Male 31-50	Female 51+	Male 51+
Calorie Level(s) Assessed		1,000	1,200	1,400, 1,600	1,600	1,800	1,800	2,200, 2,800, 3,200	2,000	2,400, 2,600, 3,000	1,800	2,200	1,600	2,000
Macronutrients														
Protein, g	RDA	13	19	19	34	34	46	52	46	56	46	56	46	56
Protein, % kcal	AMDR	5-20	10-30	10-30	10-30	10-30	10-30	10-30	10-35	10-35	10-35	10-35	10-35	10-35
Carbohydrate, g	RDA	130	130	130	130	130	130	130	130	130	130	130	130	130
Carbohydrate, % kcal	AMDR	45-65	45-65	45-65	45-65	45-65	45-65	45-65	45-65	45-65	45-65	45-65	45-65	45-65
Dietary Fiber, g	14 g/ 1,000 kcal	14	16.8	19.6	22.4	25.2	25.2	30.8	28	33.6	25.2	30.8	22.4	28
Added Sugars, % kcal	DGA	<10%	<10%	<10%	<10%	<10%	<10%	<10%	<10%	<10%	<10%	<10%	<10%	<10%
Total Fat, % kcal	AMDR	30-40	25-35	25-35	25-35	25-35	25-35	25-35	20-35	20-35	20-35	20-35	20-35	20-35
Saturated Fat, % kcal	DGA	<10%	<10%	<10%	<10%	<10%	<10%	<10%	<10%	<10%	<10%	<10%	<10%	<10%
Linoleic Acid, g	AI	7	10	10	10	12	11	16	12	17	12	17	11	14
Linolenic Acid, g	AI	0.7	0.9	0.9	1	1.2	1.1	1.6	1.1	1.6	1.1	1.6	1.1	1.6

	Source of Goal[a]	Child 1-3	Female 4-8	Male 4-8	Female 9-13	Male 9-13	Female 14-18	Male 14-18	Female 19-30	Male 19-30	Female 31-50	Male 31-50	Female 51+	Male 51+
Calorie Level(s) Assessed		1,000	1,200	1,400, 1,600	1,600	1,800	1,800	2,200, 2,800, 3,200	2,000	2,400, 2,600, 3,000	1,800	2,200	1,600	2,000
Minerals														
Calcium, mg	RDA	700	1,000	1,000	1,300	1,300	1,300	1,300	1,000	1,000	1,000	1,000	1,200	1,000[b]
Iron, mg	RDA	7	10	10	8	8	15	11	18	8	18	8	8	8
Magnesium, mg	RDA	80	130	130	240	240	360	410	310	400	320	420	320	420
Phosphorus, mg	RDA	460	500	500	1,250	1,250	1,250	1,250	700	700	700	700	700	700
Potassium, mg	AI	3,000	3,800	3,800	4,500	4,500	4,700	4,700	4,700	4,700	4,700	4,700	4,700	4,700
Sodium, mg	UL	1,500	1,900	1,900	2,200	2,200	2,300	2,300	2,300	2,300	2,300	2,300	2,300	2,300
Zinc, mg	RDA	3	5	5	8	8	9	11	8	11	8	11	8	11
Copper, mcg	RDA	340	440	440	700	700	890	890	900	900	900	900	900	900
Manganese, mg	AI	1.2	1.5	1.5	1.6	1.9	1.6	2.2	1.8	2.3	1.8	2.3	1.8	2.3
Selenium, mcg	RDA	20	30	30	40	40	55	55	55	55	55	55	55	55
Vitamins														
Vitamin A, mg RAE	RDA	300	400	400	600	600	700	900	700	900	700	900	700	900
Vitamin E, mg AT	RDA	6	7	7	11	11	15	15	15	15	15	15	15	15
Vitamin D, IU	RDA	600	600	600	600	600	600	600	600	600	600	600	600[c]	600[c]
Vitamin C, mg	RDA	15	25	25	45	45	65	75	75	90	75	90	75	90
Thiamin, mg	RDA	0.5	0.6	0.6	0.9	0.9	1	1.2	1.1	1.2	1.1	1.2	1.1	1.2
Riboflavin, mg	RDA	0.5	0.6	0.6	0.9	0.9	1	1.3	1.1	1.3	1.1	1.3	1.1	1.3
Niacin, mg	RDA	6	8	8	12	12	14	16	14	16	14	16	14	16
Vitamin B_6, mg	RDA	0.5	0.6	0.6	1	1	1.2	1.3	1.3	1.3	1.3	1.3	1.5	1.7
Vitamin B_{12}, mcg	RDA	0.9	1.2	1.2	1.8	1.8	2.4	2.4	2.4	2.4	2.4	2.4	2.4	2.4
Choline, mg	AI	200	250	250	375	375	400	550	425	550	425	550	425	550
Vitamin K, mcg	AI	30	55	55	60	60	75	75	90	120	90	120	90	120
Folate, mcg DFE	RDA	150	200	200	300	300	400	400	400	400	400	400	400	400

[a] RDA = Recommended Dietary Allowance, AI = Adequate Intake, UL = Tolerable Upper Intake Level, AMDR = Acceptable Macronutrient Distribution Range, DGA = *2015-2020 Dietary Guidelines* recommended limit; 14 g fiber per 1,000 kcal = basis for AI for fiber.

[b] Calcium RDA for males ages 71+ years is 1,200 mg.

[c] Vitamin D RDA for males and females ages 71+ years is 800 IU.

SOURCES: Institute of Medicine. Dietary Reference Intakes: The essential guide to nutrient requirements. Washington (DC): The National Academies Press; 2006.

Institute of Medicine. Dietary Reference Intakes for Calcium and Vitamin D. Washington (DC): The National Academies Press; 2010.

Appendix 8.

Federal Resources for Information on Nutrition & Physical Activity

Federal Nutrition & Physical Activity Resources

The following Federal Government resources provide reliable, science-based information on nutrition and physical activity, as well as an evolving array of tools to facilitate Americans' adoption of healthy choices.

Dietary Guidelines for Americans	www.dietaryguidelines.gov
Physical Activity Guidelines for Americans	www.health.gov/paguidelines
MyPlate	www.choosemyplate.gov
SuperTracker	www.supertracker.usda.gov
U.S. Department of Health and Human Services	www.hhs.gov
Office of Disease Prevention and Health Promotion	www.health.gov
Healthy People	www.healthypeople.gov
Healthfinder	www.healthfinder.gov
Food and Drug Administration	www.fda.gov

Centers for Disease Control and Prevention	www.cdc.gov
National Institutes of Health	www.nih.gov
Rethinking Drinking Alcoholic Beverage Calculators	http://rethinkingdrinking.niaaa.nih.gov/ToolsResources/CalculatorsMain.asp
President's Council on Fitness, Sports & Nutrition	www.fitness.gov
U.S. Department of Agriculture (USDA)	www.usda.gov
Center for Nutrition Policy and Promotion	www.cnpp.usda.gov
Food and Nutrition Service	www.fns.usda.gov
Food and Nutrition Information Center	http://fnic.nal.usda.gov
National Institute of Food and Agriculture	www.nifa.usda.gov
Let's Move!	www.letsmove.gov
U.S. National Physical Activity Plan[a]	www.physicalactivityplan.org

[a] Note: The U.S. National Physical Activity Plan is not a product of the Federal Government. However, a number of Federal offices were involved in the development of the Plan.

Appendix 9.

Alcohol

If alcohol is consumed, it should be in moderation—up to one drink per day for women and up to two drinks per day for men—and only by adults of legal drinking age. For those who choose to drink, moderate alcohol consumption can be incorporated into the calorie limits of most healthy eating patterns. The *Dietary Guidelines* does not recommend that individuals who do not drink alcohol start drinking for any reason; however, it does recommend that all foods and beverages consumed be accounted for within healthy eating patterns. Alcohol is not a component of the USDA Food Patterns. Thus, if alcohol is consumed, the calories from alcohol should be accounted for so that the limits on calories for other uses and total calories are not exceeded (see the Other Dietary Components section of Chapter 1. Key Elements of Healthy Eating Patterns for further discussion of limits on alcohol and calories for other uses within healthy eating patterns).

For the purposes of evaluating amounts of alcohol that may be consumed, the *Dietary Guidelines* includes drink-equivalents (**Table A9-1**). One alcoholic drink-equivalent is described as containing 14 g (0.6 fl oz) of pure alcohol.[1] The following are reference beverages that are one alcoholic drink-equivalent: 12 fluid ounces of regular beer (5% alcohol), 5 fluid ounces of wine (12% alcohol), or 1.5 fluid ounces of 80 proof distilled spirits (40% alcohol).[2]

Packaged (e.g., canned beer, bottled wine) and mixed beverages (e.g., margarita, rum and soda, mimosa, sangria) vary in alcohol content. For this reason it is important to determine how many alcoholic drink-equivalents are in the beverage and limit intake. **Table A9-1** lists reference beverages that are one drink-equivalent and provides examples of alcoholic drink-equivalents in other alcoholic beverages.

When determining the number of drink-equivalents in an alcoholic beverage, the variability in alcohol content and portion size must be considered together. As an example, the amount of alcohol in a beer may be higher than 5 percent and, thus, 12 ounces would be greater than one drink-equivalent. In addition to the alcohol content, the portion size may be many times larger than the reference beverage. For example, portion sizes for beer may be higher than 12 ounces and, thus, even if the alcohol content is 5 percent, the beverage would be greater than one drink-equivalent (see **Table A9-1** for additional examples). The same is true for wine and mixed drinks with distilled spirits.

Alcoholic Beverages & Calories

Alcoholic beverages may contain calories from both alcohol and other ingredients. If they are consumed, the contributions from calories from alcohol and other dietary components (e.g., added sugars, solid fats) from alcoholic beverages should be within the various limits of healthy eating patterns described in Chapter 1. One drink-equivalent contains 14 grams of pure alcohol, which contributes 98 calories to the beverage. The total calories in a beverage may be more than those from alcohol alone, depending on the type, brand, ingredients, and portion size. For example, 12 ounces of regular beer (5% alcohol) may have about 150 calories, 5 ounces of wine (12% alcohol) may have about 120 calories, and 7 ounces of a rum (40% alcohol) and cola may have about 155 calories, each with 98 calories coming from pure alcohol.[3]

Excessive Drinking

In comparison to moderate alcohol consumption, high-risk drinking is the consumption of 4 or more drinks on any day or 8 or more drinks per week for women and 5 or more drinks on any day or 15 or more drinks per week for men.

---

[1] Bowman SA, Clemens JC, Friday JE, Thoerig RC, and Moshfegh AJ. 2014. Food Patterns Equivalents Database 2011-12: Methodology and User Guide [Online]. Food Surveys Research Group, Beltsville Human Nutrition Research Center, Agricultural Research Service, U.S. Department of Agriculture, Beltsville, Maryland. Available at: http://www.ars. usda.gov/nea/bhnrc/fsrg. Accessed November 3, 2015. For additional information see the National Institute on Alcohol Abuse and Alcoholism (NIAAA) webpage available at: http://rethinkingdrinking.niaaa.nih.gov/.

[2] Drink-equivalents are not intended to serve as a standard drink definition for regulatory purposes.

[3] Calorie values are estimates, as different brands and types of beverages differ in ingredients and portion sizes and vary in their actual calorie content. For calculators to evaluate the calorie and alcohol content of alcoholic beverages, see: National Institute on Alcohol Abuse and Alcoholism (NIAAA). National Institutes of Health. Rethinking drinking, alcohol, and your health. Calculators. Available at: http://rethinkingdrinking.niaaa.nih.gov/ToolsResources/CalculatorsMain.asp. Accessed September 14, 2015.

Table A9-1.

Alcoholic Drink-Equivalents[a] of Select Beverages

Drink Description	Drink-Equivalents[b]
Beer, Beer Coolers, & Malt Beverages	
12 fl oz at 4.2% Alcohol[c]	0.8
12 fl oz at 5% Alcohol (Reference Beverage)	1
16 fl oz at 5% Alcohol	1.3
12 fl oz at 7% Alcohol	1.4
12 fl oz at 9% Alcohol	1.8
Wine	
5 fl oz at 12% Alcohol (Reference Beverage)	1
9 fl oz at 12% Alcohol	1.8
5 fl oz at 15% Alcohol	1.3
5 fl oz at 17% Alcohol	1.4
Distilled Spirits	
1.5 fl oz 80 Proof Distilled Spirits (40% Alcohol) (Reference Beverage)	1
Mixed Drink With More Than 1.5 fl oz 80 Proof Distilled Spirits (40% Alcohol)	> 1[d]

[a] One alcoholic drink-equivalent is defined as containing 14 grams (0.6 fl oz) of pure alcohol. The following are reference beverages that are one alcoholic drink-equivalent: 12 fluid ounces of regular beer (5% alcohol), 5 fluid ounces of wine (12% alcohol), or 1.5 fluid ounces of 80 proof distilled spirits (40% alcohol). Drink-equivalents are not intended to serve as a standard drink definition for regulatory purposes.

[b] To calculate drink-equivalents, multiply the volume in ounces by the alcohol content in percent and divide by 0.6 ounces of alcohol per drink-equivalent. For example: 16 fl oz beer at 5% alcohol: (16 fl oz)(0.05)/0.6 fl oz = 1.3 drink-equivalents.

[c] Light beer represents a substantial proportion of alcoholic beverages consumed in the United States. Light beer is approximately 4.2% alcohol or 0.8 alcoholic drink-equivalents in 12 fluid ounces.

[d] Depending on factors, such as the type of spirits and the recipe, one mixed drink can contain a variable number of drink-equivalents.

Binge drinking is the consumption within about 2 hours of 4 or more drinks for women and 5 or more drinks for men.

Excessive alcohol consumption—which includes binge drinking (4 or more drinks for women and 5 or more drinks for men within about 2 hours); heavy drinking (8 or more drinks a week for women and 15 or more drinks a week for men); and any drinking by pregnant women or those under 21 years of age—has no benefits. Excessive drinking is responsible for 88,000 deaths in the United States each year, including 1 in 10 deaths among working age adults (age 20-64 years). In 2006, the estimated economic cost to the United States of excessive drinking was $224 billion.[4] Binge drinking accounts for over half of the deaths and three-fourths of the economic costs due to excessive drinking.[1],[5]

Excessive drinking increases the risk of many chronic diseases and violence[6] and, over time, can impair short- and long-term cognitive function.[7] Over 90 percent of U.S. adults who drink excessively report binge drinking, and about 90 percent of the alcohol consumed by youth under 21 years of age in the United States is in the form of binge drinks. Binge drinking is associated with a wide range of health and social problems, including sexually transmitted diseases, unintended pregnancy, accidental injuries, and violent crime.[8]

Those Who Should Not Consume Alcohol

Many individuals should not consume alcohol, including individuals who are taking certain over-the-counter or prescription medications or who have certain medical conditions, those who are recovering from alcoholism or are unable to control the amount they drink, and anyone younger than age 21 years. Individuals should not drink if they are driving, planning to drive, or are participating in other activities requiring skill, coordination, and alertness.[9]

Women who are or who may be pregnant should not drink. Drinking during pregnancy, especially in the first few months of pregnancy, may result in negative behavioral or neurological consequences in the offspring. No safe level of alcohol consumption during pregnancy has been established.[10] Women who are breastfeeding should consult with their health care provider regarding alcohol consumption.[11]

Alcohol & Caffeine

Mixing alcohol and caffeine is not generally recognized as safe by the FDA.[12] People who mix alcohol and caffeine may drink more alcohol and become more intoxicated than they realize, increasing the risk of alcohol-related adverse events. Caffeine does not change blood alcohol content levels, and thus, does not reduce the risk of harms associated with drinking alcohol.[13]

[4] Stahre M, Roeber J, Kanny D, Brewer RD, Zhang X. Contribution of excessive alcohol consumption to deaths and years of potential life lost in the United States. *Prev Chronic Dis* 2014;11:130293.

[5] Bouchery EE, Harwood HJ, Sacks JJ, Simon CJ, Brewer RD. Economic costs of excessive alcohol consumption in the United States, 2006. *Am J Prev Med.* 2011;41:516–24.

[6] For more information, see: Centers for Disease Control and Prevention. Alcohol use and your health. Available at: http://www.cdc.gov/alcohol/fact-sheets/alcohol-use.htm. Accessed August 26, 2015.

[7] For more information, see: National Institute on Alcohol Abuse and Alcoholism (NIAAA). National Institutes of Health. Alcohol's effects on the body. Available at: http://www.niaaa.nih.gov/alcohol-health/alcohols-effects-body. Accessed August 26, 2015.

[8] For more information, see: Centers for Disease Control and Prevention. Fact sheets - Binge drinking. January 16, 2014. [Updated October 16, 2015.] Available at: http://www.cdc.gov/alcohol/fact-sheets/binge-drinking.htm. Accessed August 26, 2015.

[9] For more information, see: Centers for Disease Control and Prevention. Alcohol use and your health. Available at: http://www.cdc.gov/alcohol/fact-sheets/alcohol-use.htm. Accessed August26, 2015.

[10] For more information, see: Centers for Disease Control and Prevention. What you should know about alcohol and pregnancy. August 28, 2014. Available at: http://www.cdc.gov/features/alcoholandpregnancy/. Accessed August 26, 2015.

[11] Section on Breastfeeding, American Academy of Pediatrics. AAP Policy Statement: Breastfeeding and the use of human milk. *Pediatrics* 2012;129(3):e827-e841. Available at: www.pediatrics.org/cgi/doi/10.1542/peds.2011-3552. Accessed September 15, 2015.

[12] For more information, see: Food and Drug Administration. Update on caffeinated alcoholic beverages. [Updated November 24, 2010.] Available at: http://www.fda.gov/NewsEvents/PublicHealthFocus/ucm234900.htm. Accessed September 16, 2015.

[13] For more information regarding caffeine and alcohol, see CDC's Alcohol and Public Health webpage. Available at: http://www.cdc.gov/alcohol/fact-sheets/caffeine-and-alcohol.htm. Accessed August 26, 2015.

Appendix 10.

Food Sources of Potassium

Potassium: Food Sources Ranked by Amounts of Potassium & Energy per Standard Food Portions & per 100 Grams of Foods

Food	Standard Portion Size	Calories in Standard Portion[a]	Potassium in Standard Portion (mg)[a]	Calories per 100 grams[a]	Potassium per 100 grams (mg)[a]
Potato, Baked, Flesh & Skin	1 medium	163	941	94	544
Prune Juice, Canned	1 cup	182	707	71	276
Carrot Juice, Canned	1 cup	94	689	40	292
Passion-Fruit Juice, Yellow or Purple	1 cup	126-148	687	51-60	278
Tomato Paste, Canned	¼ cup	54	669	82	1,014
Beet Greens, Cooked from Fresh	½ cup	19	654	27	909
Adzuki Beans, Cooked	½ cup	147	612	128	532
White Beans, Canned	½ cup	149	595	114	454
Plain Yogurt, Nonfat	1 cup	127	579	56	255
Tomato Puree	½ cup	48	549	38	439
Sweet Potato, Baked in Skin	1 medium	103	542	90	475
Salmon, Atlantic, Wild, Cooked	3 ounces	155	534	182	628

Potassium: Food Sources Ranked by Amounts of Potassium & Energy per Standard Food Portions & per 100 Grams of Foods

Food	Standard Portion Size	Calories in Standard Portion[a]	Potassium in Standard Portion (mg)[a]	Calories per 100 grams[a]	Potassium per 100 grams (mg)[a]
Clams, Canned	3 ounces	121	534	142	628
Pomegranate Juice	1 cup	134	533	54	214
Plain Yogurt, Low-Fat	8 ounces	143	531	63	234
Tomato Juice, Canned	1 cup	41	527	17	217
Orange Juice, Fresh	1 cup	112	496	45	200
Soybeans, Green, Cooked	½ cup	127	485	141	539
Chard, Swiss, Cooked	½ cup	18	481	20	549
Lima Beans, Cooked	½ cup	108	478	115	508
Mackerel, Various Types, Cooked	3 ounces	114-171	443-474	134-201	521-558
Vegetable Juice, Canned	1 cup	48	468	19	185
Chili with Beans, Canned	½ cup	144	467	112	365
Great Northern Beans, Canned	½ cup	150	460	114	351
Yam, Cooked	½ cup	79	456	116	670
Halibut, Cooked	3 ounces	94	449	111	528
Tuna, Yellowfin, Cooked	3 ounces	111	448	130	527
Acorn Squash, Cooked	½ cup	58	448	56	437

Food	Standard Portion Size	Calories in Standard Portion[a]	Potassium in Standard Portion (mg)[a]	Calories per 100 grams[a]	Potassium per 100 grams (mg)[a]
Snapper, Cooked	3 ounces	109	444	128	522
Soybeans, Mature, Cooked	½ cup	149	443	173	515
Tangerine Juice, Fresh	1 cup	106	440	43	178
Pink Beans, Cooked	½ cup	126	430	149	508
Chocolate Milk (1%, 2% & Whole)	1 cup	178-208	418-425	71-83	167-170
Amaranth Leaves, Cooked	½ cup	14	423	21	641
Banana	1 medium	105	422	89	358
Spinach, Cooked from Fresh or Canned	½ cup	21-25	370-419	23	346-466
Black Turtle Beans, Cooked	½ cup	121	401	130	433
Peaches, Dried, Uncooked	¼ cup	96	399	239	996
Prunes, Stewed	½ cup	133	398	107	321
Rockfish, Pacific, Cooked	3 ounces	93	397	109	467
Rainbow Trout, Wild or Farmed, Cooked	3 ounces	128-143	381-383	150-168	448-450
Skim Milk (Nonfat)	1 cup	83	382	34	156
Refried Beans, Canned, Traditional	½ cup	106	380	89	319
Apricots, Dried, Uncooked	¼ cup	78	378	241	1162
Pinto Beans, Cooked	½ cup	123	373	143	436

Potassium: Food Sources Ranked by Amounts of Potassium & Energy per Standard Food Portions & per 100 Grams of Foods

Food	Standard Portion Size	Calories in Standard Portion[a]	Potassium in Standard Portion (mg)[a]	Calories per 100 grams[a]	Potassium per 100 grams (mg)[a]
Lentils, Cooked	½ cup	115	365	116	369
Avocado	½ cup	120	364	160	485
Tomato Sauce, Canned	½ cup	30	364	24	297
Plantains, Slices, Cooked	½ cup	89	358	116	465
Kidney Beans, Cooked	½ cup	113	357	127	403
Navy Beans, Cooked	½ cup	128	354	140	389

[a] Source: U.S Department of Agriculture, Agricultural Research Service, Nutrient Data Laboratory. 2014. USDA National Nutrient Database for Standard Reference, Release 27. Available at: http://www.ars.usda.gov/nutrientdata.

Appendix 11.

Food Sources of Calcium

Table A11-1.

Calcium: Food Sources Ranked by Amounts of Calcium & Energy per Standard Food Portions & per 100 Grams of Foods

Food	Standard Portion Size	Calories in Standard Portion[a]	Calcium in Standard Portion (mg)[a]	Calories per 100 grams[a]	Calcium per 100 grams (mg)[a]
Fortified Ready-to-Eat Cereals (Various)[b]	¾-1¼ cup	70-197	137-1,000	234-394	455-3,333
Pasteurized Processed American Cheese	2 ounces	210	593	371	1,045
Parmesan Cheese, Hard	1.5 ounces	167	503	392	1,184
Plain Yogurt, Nonfat	8 ounces	127	452	56	199
Romano Cheese	1.5 ounces	165	452	387	1,064
Almond Milk (All Flavors)[b]	1 cup	91-120	451	38-50	188
Pasteurized Processed Swiss Cheese	2 ounces	189	438	334	772
Tofu, Raw, Regular, Prepared with Calcium Sulfate	½ cup	94	434	76	350
Gruyere Cheese	1.5 ounces	176	430	413	1,011
Plain Yogurt, Low-Fat	8 ounces	143	415	63	183
Vanilla Yogurt, Low-Fat	8 ounces	193	388	85	171

Calcium: Food Sources Ranked by Amounts of Calcium & Energy per Standard Food Portions & per 100 Grams of Foods

Food	Standard Portion Size	Calories in Standard Portion[a]	Calcium in Standard Portion (mg)[a]	Calories per 100 grams[a]	Calcium per 100 grams (mg)[a]
Pasteurized Processed American Cheese Food	2 ounces	187	387	330	682
Fruit Yogurt, Low-Fat	8 ounces	238	383	105	169
Orange Juice, Calcium Fortified[b]	1 cup	117	349	47	140
Soymilk (All Flavors)[b]	1 cup	109	340	45	140
Ricotta Cheese, Part Skim	½ cup	171	337	138	272
Swiss Cheese	1.5 ounces	162	336	380	791
Evaporated Milk	½ cup	170	329	135	261
Sardines, Canned in Oil, Drained	3 ounces	177	325	208	382
Provolone Cheese	1.5 ounces	149	321	351	756
Monterey Cheese	1.5 ounces	159	317	373	746
Mustard Spinach (Tendergreen), Raw	1 cup	33	315	22	210
Muenster Cheese	1.5 ounces	156	305	368	717
Low-Fat Milk (1%)	1 cup	102	305	42	125
Mozzarella Cheese, Part-Skim	1.5 ounces	128	304	301	716

Food	Standard Portion Size	Calories in Standard Portion[a]	Calcium in Standard Portion (mg)[a]	Calories per 100 grams[a]	Calcium per 100 grams (mg)[a]
Skim Milk (Nonfat)	1 cup	83	299	34	122
Reduced Fat Milk (2%)	1 cup	122	293	50	120
Colby Cheese	1.5 ounces	167	291	394	685
Low-Fat Chocolate Milk (1%)	1 cup	178	290	71	116
Cheddar Cheese	1.5 ounces	173	287	406	675
Rice Drink[b]	1 cup	113	283	47	118
Whole Buttermilk	1 cup	152	282	62	115
Whole Chocolate Milk	1 cup	208	280	83	112
Whole Milk	1 cup	149	276	61	113
Reduced Fat Chocolate Milk (2%)	1 cup	190	273	76	109
Ricotta Cheese, Whole Milk	½ cup	216	257	174	207

[a] Source: U.S Department of Agriculture, Agricultural Research Service, Nutrient Data Laboratory. 2014. USDA National Nutrient Database for Standard Reference, Release 27. Available at: http://www.ars.usda.gov/nutrientdata.

[b] Calcium fortified.

Appendix 12.

Food Sources of Vitamin D

Table A12-1.

Vitamin D: Food Sources Ranked by Amounts of Vitamin D & Energy per Standard Food Portions & per 100 Grams of Foods

Food	Standard Portion Size	Calories in Standard Portion[a]	Vitamin D in Standard Portion (µg)[a,b]	Calories per 100 grams[a]	Vitamin D per 100 grams (µg)[a,b]
Salmon, Sockeye, Canned	3 ounces	142	17.9	167	21.0
Trout, Rainbow, Farmed, Cooked	3 ounces	143	16.2	168	19.0
Salmon, Chinook, Smoked	3 ounces	99	14.5	117	17.1
Swordfish, Cooked	3 ounces	146	14.1	172	16.6
Sturgeon, Mixed Species, Smoked	3 ounces	147	13.7	173	16.1
Salmon, Pink, Canned	3 ounces	117	12.3	138	14.5
Fish Oil, Cod Liver	1 tsp	41	11.3	902	250
Cisco, Smoked	3 ounces	150	11.3	177	13.3
Salmon, Sockeye, Cooked	3 ounces	144	11.1	169	13.1
Salmon, Pink, Cooked	3 ounces	130	11.1	153	13.0
Sturgeon, Mixed Species, Cooked	3 ounces	115	11.0	135	12.9

Food	Standard Portion Size	Calories in Standard Portion[a]	Vitamin D in Standard Portion (µg)[a,b]	Calories per 100 grams[a]	Vitamin D per 100 grams (µg)[a,b]
Whitefish, Mixed Species, Smoked	3 ounces	92	10.9	108	12.8
Mackerel, Pacific & Jack, Cooked	3 ounces	171	9.7	201	11.4
Salmon, Coho, Wild, Cooked	3 ounces	118	9.6	139	11.3
Mushrooms, Portabella, Exposed to Ultraviolet Light, Grilled	½ cup	18	7.9	29	13.1
Tuna, Light, Canned in Oil, Drained	3 ounces	168	5.7	198	6.7
Halibut, Atlantic & Pacific, Cooked	3 ounces	94	4.9	111	5.8
Herring, Atlantic, Cooked	3 ounces	173	4.6	203	5.4
Sardine, Canned in Oil, Drained	3 ounces	177	4.1	208	4.8
Rockfish, Pacific, Mixed Species, Cooked	3 ounces	93	3.9	109	4.6
Whole Milk[c]	1 cup	149	3.2	61	1.3
Whole Chocolate Milk[c]	1 cup	208	3.2	83	1.3
Tilapia, Cooked	3 ounces	109	3.1	128	3.7
Flatfish (Flounder & Sole), Cooked	3 ounces	73	3.0	86	3.5
Reduced Fat Chocolate Milk (2%)[c]	1 cup	190	3.0	76	1.2

Vitamin D: Food Sources Ranked by Amounts of Vitamin D & Energy per Standard Food Portions & per 100 Grams of Foods

Food	Standard Portion Size	Calories in Standard Portion[a]	Vitamin D in Standard Portion (μg)[a,b]	Calories per 100 grams[a]	Vitamin D per 100 grams (μg)[a,b]
Yogurt (Various Types & Flavors)[c]	8 ounces	98-254	2.0-3.0	43-112	0.9-1.3
Milk (Non-Fat, 1% & 2%)[c]	1 cup	83-122	2.9	34-50	1.2
Soymilk[c]	1 cup	109	2.9	45	1.2
Low-Fat Chocolate Milk (1%)[c]	1 cup	178	2.8	71	1.1
Fortified Ready-to-Eat Cereals (Various)[c]	⅓-1¼ cup	74-247	0.2-2.5	248-443	0.8-8.6
Orange Juice, Fortified[c]	1 cup	117	2.5	47	1.0
Almond Milk (All Flavors)[c]	1 cup	91-120	2.4	38-50	1.0
Rice Drink[c]	1 cup	113	2.4	47	1.0
Pork, Cooked (Various Cuts)	3 ounces	122-390	0.2-2.2	143-459	0.2-2.6
Mushrooms, Morel, Raw	½ cup	10	1.7	31	5.1
Margarine (Various)[c]	1 Tbsp	75-100	1.5	533-717	10.7
Mushrooms, Chanterelle, Raw	½ cup	10	1.4	38	5.3
Egg, Hard-Boiled	1 large	78	1.1	155	2.2

[a] Source: U.S Department of Agriculture, Agricultural Research Service, Nutrient Data Laboratory. 2014. USDA National Nutrient Database for Standard Reference, Release 27. Available at: http://www.ars.usda.gov/nutrientdata.

[b] 1 μg of vitamin D is equivalent to 40 IU.

[c] Vitamin D fortified.

Appendix 13.

Food Sources of Dietary Fiber

Table A13-1.

Dietary Fiber: Food Sources Ranked by Amounts of Dietary Fiber & Energy per Standard Food Portions & per 100 Grams of Foods

Food	Standard Portion Size	Calories in Standard Portion[a]	Dietary Fiber in Standard Portion (g)[a]	Calories per 100 grams[a]	Dietary Fiber per 100 grams (g)[a]
High Fiber Bran Ready-to-Eat Cereal	½-¾ cup	60-81	9.1-14.3	200-260	29.3-47.5
Navy Beans, Cooked	½ cup	127	9.6	140	10.5
Small White Beans, Cooked	½ cup	127	9.3	142	10.4
Yellow Beans, Cooked	½ cup	127	9.2	144	10.4
Shredded Wheat Ready-to-Eat Cereal (Various)	1-1¼ cup	155-220	5.0-9.0	321-373	9.6-15.0
Cranberry (Roman) Beans, Cooked	½ cup	120	8.9	136	10.0
Adzuki Beans, Cooked	½ cup	147	8.4	128	7.3
French Beans, Cooked	½ cup	114	8.3	129	9.4
Split Peas, Cooked	½ cup	114	8.1	116	8.3
Chickpeas, Canned	½ cup	176	8.1	139	6.4
Lentils, Cooked	½ cup	115	7.8	116	7.9

Dietary Fiber: Food Sources Ranked by Amounts of Dietary Fiber & Energy per Standard Food Portions & per 100 Grams of Foods

Food	Standard Portion Size	Calories in Standard Portion[a]	Dietary Fiber in Standard Portion (g)[a]	Calories per 100 grams[a]	Dietary Fiber per 100 grams (g)[a]
Pinto Beans, Cooked	½ cup	122	7.7	143	9.0
Black Turtle Beans, Cooked	½ cup	120	7.7	130	8.3
Mung Beans, Cooked	½ cup	106	7.7	105	7.6
Black Beans, Cooked	½ cup	114	7.5	132	8.7
Artichoke, Globe or French, Cooked	½ cup	45	7.2	53	8.6
Lima Beans, Cooked	½ cup	108	6.6	115	7.0
Great Northern Beans, Canned	½ cup	149	6.4	114	4.9
White Beans, Canned	½ cup	149	6.3	114	4.8
Kidney Beans, All Types, Cooked	½ cup	112	5.7	127	6.4
Pigeon Peas, Cooked	½ cup	102	5.6	121	6.7
Cowpeas, Cooked	½ cup	99	5.6	116	6.5
Wheat Bran Flakes Ready-to-Eat Cereal (Various)	¾ cup	90-98	4.9-5.5	310-328	16.9-18.3
Pear, Raw	1 medium	101	5.5	57	3.1
Pumpkin Seeds, Whole, Roasted	1 ounce	126	5.2	446	18.4

Food	Standard Portion Size	Calories in Standard Portion[a]	Dietary Fiber in Standard Portion (g)[a]	Calories per 100 grams[a]	Dietary Fiber per 100 grams (g)[a]
Baked Beans, Canned, Plain	½ cup	119	5.2	94	4.1
Soybeans, Cooked	½ cup	149	5.2	173	6.0
Plain Rye Wafer Crackers	2 wafers	73	5.0	334	22.9
Avocado	½ cup	120	5.0	160	6.7
Broadbeans (Fava Beans), Cooked	½ cup	94	4.6	110	5.4
Pink Beans, Cooked	½ cup	126	4.5	149	5.3
Apple, with Skin	1 medium	95	4.4	52	2.4
Green Peas, Cooked (Fresh, Frozen, Canned)	½ cup	59-67	3.5-4.4	69-84	4.1-5.5
Refried Beans, Canned	½ cup	107	4.4	90	3.7
Chia Seeds, Dried	1 Tbsp	58	4.1	486	34.4
Bulgur, Cooked	½ cup	76	4.1	83	4.5
Mixed Vegetables, Cooked from Frozen	½ cup	59	4.0	65	4.4
Raspberries	½ cup	32	4.0	52	6.5
Blackberries	½ cup	31	3.8	43	5.3
Collards, Cooked	½ cup	32	3.8	33	4.0
Soybeans, Green, Cooked	½ cup	127	3.8	141	4.2
Prunes, Stewed	½ cup	133	3.8	107	3.1

Table A13-1. *(continued...)*

Dietary Fiber: Food Sources Ranked by Amounts of Dietary Fiber & Energy per Standard Food Portions & per 100 Grams of Foods

Food	Standard Portion Size	Calories in Standard Portion[a]	Dietary Fiber in Standard Portion (g)[a]	Calories per 100 grams[a]	Dietary Fiber per 100 grams (g)[a]
Sweet Potato, Baked in Skin	1 medium	103	3.8	90	3.3
Figs, Dried	¼ cup	93	3.7	249	9.8
Pumpkin, Canned	½ cup	42	3.6	34	2.9
Potato, Baked, with Skin	1 medium	163	3.6	94	2.1
Popcorn, Air-Popped	3 cups	93	3.5	387	14.5
Almonds	1 ounce	164	3.5	579	12.5
Pears, Dried	¼ cup	118	3.4	262	7.5
Whole Wheat Spaghetti, Cooked	½ cup	87	3.2	124	4.5
Parsnips, Cooked	½ cup	55	3.1	71	4.0
Sunflower Seed Kernels, Dry Roasted	1 ounce	165	3.1	582	11.1
Orange	1 medium	69	3.1	49	2.2
Banana	1 medium	105	3.1	89	2.6
Guava	1 fruit	37	3.0	68	5.4
Oat Bran Muffin	1 small	178	3.0	270	4.6
Pearled Barley, Cooked	½ cup	97	3.0	123	3.8

Food	Standard Portion Size	Calories in Standard Portion[a]	Dietary Fiber in Standard Portion (g)[a]	Calories per 100 grams[a]	Dietary Fiber per 100 grams (g)[a]
Winter Squash, Cooked	½ cup	38	2.9	37	2.8
Dates	¼ cup	104	2.9	282	8.0
Pistachios, Dry Roasted	1 ounce	161	2.8	567	9.9
Pecans, Oil Roasted	1 ounce	203	2.7	715	9.5
Hazelnuts or Filberts	1 ounce	178	2.7	628	9.7
Peanuts, Oil Roasted	1 ounce	170	2.7	599	9.4
Whole Wheat Paratha Bread	1 ounce	92	2.7	326	9.6
Quinoa, Cooked	½ cup	111	2.6	120	2.8

[a] Source: U.S Department of Agriculture, Agricultural Research Service, Nutrient Data Laboratory. 2014. USDA National Nutrient Database for Standard Reference, Release 27. Available at: http://www.ars.usda.gov/nutrientdata.

Appendix 14.
Food Safety Principles & Guidance

An important part of healthy eating is keeping foods safe. It is estimated that foodborne illness affects about 1 in 6 Americans (or 48 million people), leading to 128,000 hospitalizations and 3,000 deaths every year.[1] Food may be handled numerous times as it moves from the farm to homes. Individuals in their own homes can reduce contaminants and help keep food safe to eat by following safe food handling practices. Four basic food safety principles work together to reduce the risk of foodborne illness—Clean, Separate, Cook, and Chill. These four principles are the cornerstones of Fight BAC!®, a national food safety education campaign aimed at consumers.

Clean

Microbes, such as bacteria and viruses, can be spread throughout the kitchen and get onto hands, cutting boards, utensils, countertops, reusable grocery bags, and foods. This is called "cross-contamination." Hand washing is important to prevent contamination of food with microbes from raw animal products (e.g., raw seafood, meat, poultry, and eggs) and from people (e.g., cold, flu, and Staph infections). Frequent cleaning of surfaces is essential in preventing cross-contamination. To reduce microbes and contaminants from foods, all produce, regardless of where it was grown or purchased, should be thoroughly rinsed. This is particularly important for produce that will be eaten raw.

[1] http://www.cdc.gov/foodborneburden/. Accessed June 1, 2015.

Hands

Hands should be washed before and after preparing food, especially after handling raw seafood, meat, poultry, or eggs, and before eating. In addition, hand washing is recommended after going to the bathroom, changing diapers, coughing or sneezing, tending to someone who is sick or injured, touching animals, and handling garbage. Hands should be washed using soap and water. Soaps with antimicrobial agents are not needed for consumer hand washing, and their use over time can lead to growth of microbes resistant to these agents. Alcohol-based (≥ 60%), rinse-free hand sanitizers should be used when hand washing with soap is not possible. Hand sanitizers are not as effective when hands are visibly dirty or greasy.

Wash Hands With Soap & Water

- Wet hands with clean running water (warm or cold), turn off tap, and apply soap.

- Rub hands together to make lather and scrub the back of hands, between fingers, and under nails for at least 20 seconds. If you need a timer you can hum the "happy birthday" song from beginning to end twice.

- Rinse hands well under running water.

- Dry hands using a clean towel or air dry them.

Surfaces

Surfaces should be washed with hot, soapy water. A solution of 1 tablespoon of unscented, liquid chlorine bleach per gallon of water can be used to sanitize surfaces. All kitchen surfaces should be kept clean, including tables, countertops, sinks, utensils, cutting boards, and appliances. For example, the insides of microwaves easily become soiled with food, allowing microbes to grow. They should be cleaned often.

Keep Appliances Clean

- At least once a week, throw out refrigerated foods that should no longer be eaten.

- Cooked leftovers should be discarded after 4 days; raw poultry and ground meats, 1 to 2 days.

- Wipe up spills immediately—clean food-contact surfaces often.

- Clean the inside and the outside of appliances. Pay particular attention to buttons and handles where cross-contamination to hands can occur.

Foods

Vegetables & Fruits. All produce, regardless of where it was grown or purchased, should be thoroughly rinsed. However, any precut packaged items, like lettuce or baby carrots, are labeled as prewashed and ready-to-eat. These products can be eaten without further rinsing.

- Rinse fresh vegetables and fruits under running water just before eating, cutting, or cooking.

- Do not use soap or detergent to clean produce; commercial produce washes are not needed.

- Even if you plan to peel or cut the produce before eating, it is still important to thoroughly rinse it first to prevent microbes from transferring from the outside to the inside of the produce.

- Scrub the skin or rind of firm produce, such as melons and cucumbers, with a clean produce brush while you rinse it.

- Dry produce with a clean cloth towel or paper towel to further reduce bacteria that may be present. Wet produce can allow remaining microbes to multiply faster.

Seafood, Meat, & Poultry. Raw seafood, meat, and poultry should not be rinsed. Bacteria in these raw juices can spread to other foods, utensils, and surfaces, leading to foodborne illness.

Separate

Separating foods that are ready-to-eat from those that are raw or that might otherwise contain harmful microbes is key to preventing foodborne illness. Attention should be given to separating foods at every step of food handling, from purchase to preparation to serving.

Separate Foods When Shopping

- Place raw seafood, meat, and poultry in plastic bags. Separate them from other foods in your grocery cart and bags.

- Store raw seafood, meat, and poultry below ready-to-eat foods in your refrigerator.

- Clean reusable grocery bags regularly. Wash canvas and cloth bags in the washing machine and wash plastic reusable bags with hot, soapy water.

Separate Foods When Preparing & Serving Food

- Always use a clean cutting board for fresh produce and a separate one for raw seafood, meat, and poultry.

- Always use a clean plate to serve and eat food.

- Never place cooked food back on the same plate or cutting board that previously held raw food.

Cook & Chill

Seafood, meat, poultry, and egg dishes should be cooked to the recommended safe minimum internal temperature to destroy harmful microbes (see **Table A14-1**). It is not always possible to tell whether a food is safe by how it looks. A food thermometer should be used to ensure that food is safely cooked and that cooked food is held at safe temperatures until eaten. In general, the food thermometer should be placed in the thickest part of the food, not touching bone, fat, or gristle. The manufacturer's instructions should be followed for the amount of time needed to measure the temperature of foods. Food thermometers should be cleaned with hot, soapy water before and after each use.

Temperature rules also apply to microwave cooking. Microwave ovens can cook unevenly and leave "cold spots" where harmful bacteria can survive. When cooking using a microwave, foods should be stirred, rotated, and/or flipped periodically to help them cook evenly. Microwave cooking instructions on food packages always should be followed.

Keep Foods at Safe Temperatures

- Hold cold foods at 40°F or below.

- Keep hot foods at 140°F or above.

- Foods are no longer safe to eat when they have been in the danger zone of 40-140°F for more than 2 hours (1 hour if the temperature was above 90°F).

  - When shopping, the 2-hour window includes the amount of time food is in the grocery basket, car, and on the kitchen counter.

  - As soon as frozen food begins to thaw and become warmer than 40°F, any bacteria that may have been present before freezing can begin to multiply. Use one of the three safe ways to thaw foods: (1) in the refrigerator, (2) in cold water (i.e., in a leak proof bag, changing cold water every 30 minutes), or (3) in the microwave. Never thaw food on the counter. Keep your refrigerator at 40°F or below.

- Keep your freezer at 0°F or below. Monitor these temperatures with appliance thermometers.

Table A14-1.
Recommended Safe Minimum Internal Temperatures

Consumers should cook foods to the minimum internal temperatures shown below. The temperature should be measured with a clean food thermometer before removing meat from the heat source. For safety and quality, allow meat to rest for at least 3 minutes before carving or consuming. For reasons of personal preference, consumers may choose to cook meat to higher temperatures.

Food	Degrees Fahrenheit
Ground Meat & Meat Mixtures	
Beef, Pork, Veal, Lamb	160
Turkey, Chicken	165
Fresh Beef, Pork, Veal, Lamb	
Steaks, Roasts, Chops	145
Poultry	
Chicken & Turkey, Whole	165
Poultry Breasts, Roasts	165
Poultry Thighs, Wings	165
Duck & Goose	165
Stuffing (Cooked Alone or in Bird)	165
Fresh Pork	160
Ham	
Fresh Ham (Raw)	145
Pre-cooked Ham (to Reheat)	140
Eggs & Egg Dishes	
Eggs	Cook until yolk and white are firm.
Egg Dishes	160
Fresh Seafood	
Finfish	145; Cook fish until it is opaque (milky white) and flakes with a fork.
Shellfish	Cook shrimp, lobster, and scallops until they reach their appropriate color. The flesh of shrimp and lobster should be an opaque (milky white) color. Scallops should be opaque (milky white) and firm. Cook clams, mussels, and oysters until their shells open. This means that they are done. Throw away the ones that didn't open. Shucked clams and shucked oysters are fully cooked when they are opaque (milky white) and firm.
Leftovers & Casseroles	165

Risky Eating Behaviors

Harmful bacteria, viruses, and parasites usually do not change the look or smell of food. This makes it impossible for consumers to know whether food is contaminated. Consumption of raw or undercooked animal food products increases the risk of contracting a foodborne illness. Raw or undercooked foods commonly eaten in the United States include eggs (e.g., eggs with runny yolks), ground beef (e.g., undercooked hamburger), dairy (e.g., cheese made from unpasteurized milk), and seafood (e.g., raw oysters). Cooking foods to recommended safe minimum internal temperatures and consuming only pasteurized dairy products are the best ways to reduce the risk of foodborne illness from animal products. Always use pasteurized eggs or egg products when preparing foods that are made with raw eggs (e.g., eggnog, smoothies and other drinks, hollandaise sauce, ice cream, and uncooked cookie dough). Consumers who choose to eat raw seafood despite the risks should choose seafood that has been previously frozen, which will kill parasites but not harmful microbes.

Specific Populations at Increased Risk of Foodborne Illness

Some individuals, including women who are pregnant and their unborn children, young children, older adults, and individuals with weakened immune systems (such as those living with HIV infection, cancer treatment, organ transplant, or liver disease), are more susceptible than the general population to the effects of foodborne illnesses such as listeriosis and salmonellosis. The outcome of contracting a foodborne illness for these individuals can be severe or even fatal. They need to take special care to keep foods safe and to not eat foods that increase the risk of foodborne illness. Women who are pregnant, infants and young children, older adults, and people with weakened immune systems should only eat foods containing seafood, meat, poultry, or eggs that have been cooked to recommended safe minimum internal temperatures. They also should take special precautions not to consume unpasteurized (raw) juice or milk or foods made from unpasteurized milk, like some soft cheeses (e.g., Feta, queso blanco, queso fresco, Brie, Camembert cheeses, blue-veined cheeses, and Panela). They should reheat deli and luncheon meats and hot dogs to steaming hot to kill Listeria, the bacteria that causes listeriosis, and not eat raw sprouts, which also can carry harmful bacteria.

Resources for Additional Food Safety Information

Federal Food Safety Gateway: www.foodsafety.gov

Fight BAC!®: www.fightbac.org

Be Food Safe: www.befoodsafe.gov

Is It Done Yet?: www.isitdoneyet.gov

Thermy™: http://www.fsis.usda.gov/wps/portal/fsis/topics/food-safety-education/teach-others/fsis-educational-campaigns/thermy

For more information and answers to specific questions:

- Call the USDA Meat and Poultry Hotline 1-888-MPHotline (1-888-674-6854) TTY: 1-800- 256-7072. Hours: 10:00 a.m. to 4:00 p.m. Eastern time, Monday through Friday, in English and Spanish, or email: mphotline.fsis@usda.gov

- Visit "Ask Karen," FSIS's Web-based automated response system at www.fsis.usda.gov

Notes

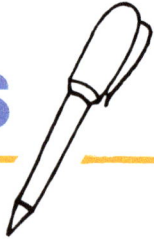
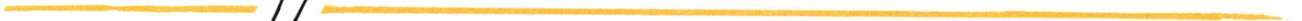

www.ingramcontent.com/pod-product-compliance
Lightning Source LLC
Chambersburg PA
CBHW080621270326
41928CB00016B/3154